Holistic Microneedling

The Manual of Natural Skin Needling

1st Edition

By Anthony Kingston (MSc)

Bright Pen

Visit us online at www.authorsonline.co.uk

A Bright Pen Book

British Library Cataloguing in Publication Data.
A catalogue record for this book is available from the
British Library.

ISBN 978 0 7552 1492 1

Authors OnLine Ltd
19 The Cinques
Gamlingay, Sandy
Bedfordshire SG19 3NU
England

This book is also available in e-book format, details of which are available
at www.authorsonline.co.uk

Notice to the Reader

This book is not intended as a substitute for the medical advice of physicians. The reader should regularly consult a physician in matters relating to his/her health and particularly with respect to any symptoms that may require diagnosis or medical attention.

Always consult a physician or other qualified health care professional properly licensed to practice health care in your region concerning any questions you may have about the information contained in this book, or any medical condition you believe you may have.

This book is current to existing regulation in the UK at the time of publishing. Requirements for approval of some protocols may differ in your local region significantly so please check with your local authorities.

This book is not meant to be a substitute for proper instruction in the use of microneedling which should be carried out by a suitably qualified practitioner.

Although the author has made every effort to ensure that the information in this book was correct at press time, the author does not assume and hereby disclaim any liability to any party for any loss, damage, or disruption caused by errors or omissions, whether such errors or omissions result from negligence, accident, or any other cause.

About the Author

Anthony Kingston completed 5 years of tertiary study in acupuncture and Chinese herbal medicine in Sydney Australia. He and his wife Kamila then travelled repeatedly to China, Malaysia and Singapore to study the Asian understanding of cosmetic skin needling. On returning to Australia they set up White Lotus Cosmetic Acupuncture the first specialist cosmetic acupuncture clinic in Australasia. This clinic became well known due to its innovative adaptions of traditional anti aging techniques to modern tastes.

During this time they began to incorporate modern microneedling or skin needling into their clinic and quickly saw the benefits of adapting this modern treatment back into a traditional philosophy of anti aging such as is found in parts of Asia.

Anthony has demonstrated many of his skin needling techniques on National television and has repeatedly written articles for a variety of general interest and scientific publications. He holds a BSc in acupuncture and complementary medicine and an MSc in herbal medicine focused on pharmacology. He currently lives in Sussex UK with his wife and young daughter.

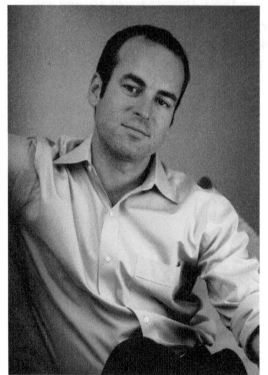

For more information about the content of the book please visit his website at www.whitelotusantiaging.com or email: info@whitelotusantiaging.com

Special thanks to Kamila and Kaia for your support and for forgiving my absence while I wrote this. I simply would not have done it without you. Thanks also to Jane Kingston for her proof reading and suggested changes. This is a better book for them. A final thanks to all my students over the years who have increased my knowledge through their own experiences.

Table of Contents

1.5mm Microneedle Roller
2.0mm Microneedle Roller
3.0mm Microneedle Roller
Dermastamp
Needle Length Reference Table

Principle 3 – Apply the Principles of Traditional Medicine to Improve Microneedling Treatments

Chapter 11 - Why Apply a Traditional Medicine System?
The Traditional Chinese Understanding of Beauty
Applying the Acupuncture Meridians to Microneedling
Individualised Treatments
Simple Steps to Apply TCM Theory to a Microneedling Treatment

Part 3 - Putting it All Together – Performing Holistic Microneedling Treatments

Chapter 12 - Prior to Treatment
Cautions and Contraindications
Skin Conditions
Medications
Cosmetic Treatments
Other Considerations
Treatment Schedule
Cleansing the Skin to be treated

Chapter 13 – Performing Microneedling Treatments
Rolling Techniques
Explanation of the Techniques
Additional Products used with the Treatments

Treatment Tinctures
Anti Aging Tincture
Scar and Stretch Marks Tincture
Cellulite Tincture
Clear Skin Tincture

Aftercare Serums
Anti Aging Aftercare Serum
Scar Aftercare Serum
Stretch Mark and Cellulite Aftercare Serum
Aftercare Hair Restoration Spray

Microneedling Techniques
Techniques for Treating the Face
Notes for Treating the Face
Techniques for Treating for the Neck
Notes for Treating the Neck
Techniques for Treating the Décolletage
Notes for Treating the Décolletage
Techniques for Treating the Hands
Notes for Treating the Hands
Techniques for Treating the Abdomen
Notes for treating the Abdomen
Techniques for Treating the Thighs
Notes for treating the Thighs
Techniques for Treating the Upper Arms
Notes for Treating the Upper Arms
Techniques for Assisting Hair Restoration
Notes for Assisting Hair Restoration
Quick Reference Table

Introduction

In the last decade several hundred thousand microneedling treatments have been performed in the western world. Yet prior to 2000 it was an unheard of practice mulling around the back pages of dry scientific trials on drug absorption. So what changed? Interestingly in an industry often driven by hype and marketing, it is the results that microneedling can produce that are really setting it apart.

The cosmetic industry has long focused on the induction, or application of collagen to the skin to achieve impressive results. To achieve these results the skin has been chemically peeled, burnt, cut, injected and scraped to name but a few. The advent of microneedling has allowed clinicians to induce large quantities of the body's own natural collagen without having to apply any of these more aggressive techniques. This has led to more affordable treatments, with lower side effects, shorter recovery times and happier clients.

Microneedling uses the body's own natural resources to produce collagen. Several other cosmetic treatments also work this way; however, all of them involve either removing or potentially burning the outer layers of the skin to reach the deeper layers where collagen production takes place. Microneedling can reach these deeper levels by creating tiny holes which heal completely within hours. The ability of microneedling to work with the body in this way, with very few side effects, makes it an obvious candidate for a genuinely natural, holistic cosmetic treatment.

The worldwide trend towards holistic and natural treatments is growing rapidly. Demand in the cosmetic industry is not exempt from this trend. The stumbling point for many natural treatments has traditionally been practicality. Short expiry dates, bad smells, the need for refrigeration and inconvenient preparations have often deterred people who would otherwise prefer natural treatments. The inability of many natural treatments to demonstrate measurable improvements has also often tarnished the industry.

Microneedling appears to be an obvious solution for this growing demand. It is simple to perform, works with the body, produces very few side effects and has strong scientific evidence and patient feedback to support it. It has the potential to be the effective alternative treatment for many clinicians and home use clients seeking more natural and effective cosmetic treatments.

Unfortunately, any drive towards creating natural microneedling treatments has largely been a victim of the wider philosophy of the cosmetic industry. As a whole the cosmetic industry has lost touch with the connection between health and beauty. As a result treatments are often designed to overcome the body's appearance rather than to work with the body's natural biological processes. Most treatments are developed in laboratories far away from any real users. This is reflected in many treatments which often view the area being treated as isolated cells which are misbehaving rather than as part of a functioning human being. Any and all attempts are made to improve the short term appearance of these cells often at the expense of wider well-being and long term appearance of the client.

The effects of this wider industry philosophy have been detrimental to microneedling in a number of ways including:

1. The use of a wide variety of synthetic and usually unnecessary compounds applied with the treatments, many producing side effects.
2. Far longer needles being used than are necessary creating unnecessary trauma at deeper levels of the skin to which the body must then allocate resources for healing
3. Heavy handed techniques being advocated encouraging excessive bleeding and trauma which necessitates the use of anaesthetics.
4. Finally a one size fits all strategy being applied to all patients regardless of need or their individual constitution and skin make up.

In order to allow microneedling to fulfil its potential as a holistic treatment it is necessary to incorporate a holistic philosophy into the treatments. This is more useful than simply advocating natural products or techniques as it influences the entire practice. Once this philosophy is established it will then automatically dictate the techniques and practices and ensure they are performed in a natural and holistic way.

Traditional Chinese Medicine is an obvious place from which to draw this philosophy as the earliest form of cosmetic skin needling was performed using acupuncture needles. This philosophy is well-established and has been refined over thousands of years.

This Traditional Chinese philosophy is very results driven as modern scientists studying acupuncture techniques are discovering. It was also however a philosophy that advocated working with the body rather than against it to achieve results. Individuals were viewed as a whole rather than as random groupings of cells. It is from systems such as this that we derive the term holistic to describe actually seeing and treating an individual as a whole person. Once this philosophy is established it creates a framework in which only practices that benefit the body as a whole while achieving results are adopted.

As Traditional Chinese Medicine already used skin needling in the form of acupuncture, incorporating microneedling into this philosophy is quite simple and very effective. It is also very easy to learn and does not require extensive training in Chinese Medicine as the modern microneedle rollers are so simple to use.

This book is the result of years of clinical practice incorporating microneedling into a specialist cosmetic acupuncture clinic. The practices developed are simple to perform and easily integrated into any cosmetic clinic. They are also often enlightening for individuals using home use rollers who have often received very little instruction in how to make the most of their microneedle rollers. The book contains more than simply a list of techniques. I have incorporated 3 core principles that can be adhered to too achieve very safe, effective microneedling treatments.

I have coined the term 'holistic microneedling' to describe these 3 core principles and the techniques and practices which are a natural progression from them. It is hoped that by providing principles as well as techniques it will provide clinicians with a holistic framework in which to apply microneedling. This can lead to more innovative techniques and the growth of the industry while retaining the focus on the whole person's well-being.

The 3 Principals of Holistic Microneedling

Principle 1 – Use Only Natural Substances During Microneedling Treatments

All substances used before, during and after the microneedling treatments have to be natural in origin. I do not include mass produced synthetic vitamins, minerals, peptides or stem cells in this category. Microneedling is known to dramatically increase the absorption of products through the skin making it very important we know exactly what is being absorbed. As the word natural is widely misused and misunderstood in our society I have developed a simple process for determining if a substance is natural and holistic and have described it in detail in later chapters.

Principle 2 – Use the Least Invasive Microneedling Techniques to Achieve the Desired Results

This is a principle which influences which needle length you choose, the length of treatment and the techniques used during treatment. In adopting microneedling the cosmetic industry has applied its existing philosophy that excessive damage to the skin is often justified for short term results. The natural progression from this attitude is the use of more and more invasive and damaging techniques to ensure quick results at any cost. To create holistic microneedling we need to use the shortest needles possible and cause the minimum trauma possible to achieve the desired results. We also need to apply very specific rolling techniques to minimise any pain or side effects caused by the treatments. To do otherwise is simply creating an unnecessary burden on the body's resources.

Principle 3 – Apply the Principals of Traditional Medicine to Improve Microneedling Treatments

The principals of traditional medicine systems such as Chinese Medicine were designed to work with the body as a whole. Excessive trauma could not be applied to one part of the body without ramifications for the rest of the body. Achieving this holistic approach to microneedling is simple to achieve when we apply the theories of Chinese Medicine and acupuncture theory to modern microneedling. This provides us with a framework in which to work and a foundation for the treatments. This principal leads us to a variety of possibilities for the use of microneedling combined with natural ingredients for therapeutic as well as cosmetic purposes.

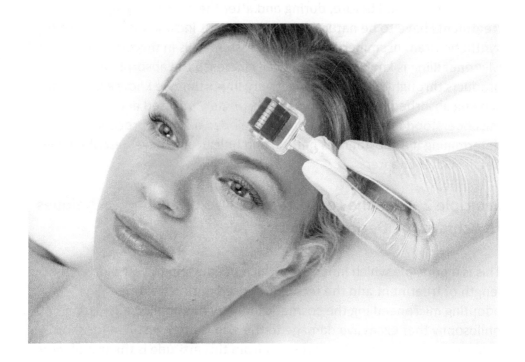

Part 1 - Background

Chapter 1 - What is Microneedling?

Working Definition of Microneedling

Microneedling in its essence is the penetration of the skin by very small needles. The microneedles are spaced very close together allowing a high number of needles to penetrate the skin in a very small area. In common usage the term has come increasingly to refer to the use of microneedle rollers to actively penetrate the skin to a certain depth in order to induce collagen or increase transdermal absorption (the absorption of products through the skin).

I am frequently asked whether the microneedles actually inject something into the skin to achieve results. The answer is no, they do increase the absorption of products applied to the skin but they do not actually inject anything. The collagen induction is produced completely naturally by the body in response to the micro trauma produced by the penetration of the needles.

Producing collagen is one of the principal aims of modern beauty treatments leading to much younger looking skin. The increase in transdermal absorption can also be of great benefit as it can allow the skin to absorb products which improve the skins appearance in much greater quantities.

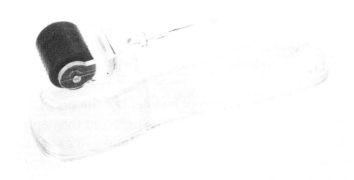

Image 1: A Modern Microneedle Roller

Different Names for Microneedling

There are many different names for microneedling in different countries. This is partly because of different routes of development but also partly due to the economic use of trademarks. Many companies have developed their own trademark for the technique as a way of differentiating themselves.

This has been further enhanced recently when one company managed to trademark the word 'dermaroller' in both Australia and the USA. Prior to this, the word dermaroller was often used as a general term for the use of microneedle rollers. These trademarks have led to the treatments continuing to be described by the word dermaroller in Europe but not in Australia or the USA.

Some of the more common names to describe the process of microneedling are Skin needling, Percutaneous Collagen Induction (PCI), Collagen Induction Therapy (CIT), Needle-dermabrasion, Derma Rolling, Dermal Needling and Multi-Trepannic Collagen Actuation.

In addition to this many of the products themselves have become so popular that the brand name has become synonymous with the treatment. These names include Roll-CIT, Lotus Roller, Dermaroller and MTS-Roller.

What is the Microneedle Roller Made From?
The Handle

The roller handle and drum are usually made from a variety of different plastic compounds depending on the quality of the particular roller. Many companies spend a lot of time advertising the quality and strength of their roller handles. This is unfortunate as any pressure great enough to break or bend the handle will have inevitably damaged the needles first and rendered the roller useless.

There are several different types of handles but the principle designs are either cylindrical or flat. In clinic I always preferred the flat handles. There are several reasons for this. The flat handle makes it easier to be sure the roller is in maximum contact with the skin. With a cylindrical handle it is easier not to have the drum of the roller parallel with the skin and so only one side of the roller (left or right) is touching the skin giving an uneven treatment. By aligning the flat roller handle parallel with the skin during treatment this is largely avoided. This is particularly important if using the roller at home as it is often hard to see if all the needles are in contact with the skin.

I also find that the flat handle acts like a suspension mechanism. This allows the roller to cross raised areas like moles without causing undue damage. One final drawback of the cylindrical handle is the container in which they arrive. It is often hard to get them out of the round cylinder without touching the sides which bends the needles on the edge of the roller before you even begin.

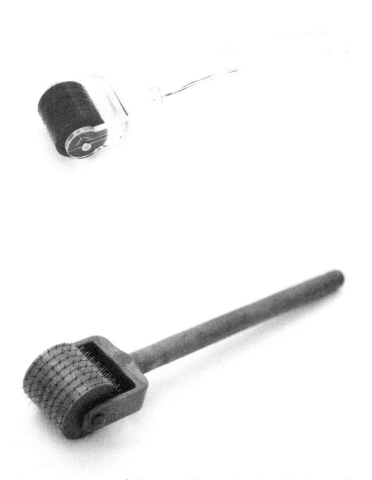

Image 2 – A Comparison of Flat Handles and Cylindrical Handles

The Microneedles
The number of needles on the roller varies but most now contain 192. The sharper the needle the less painful the treatment will be as the needles pass smoothly through the skin. This sounds counter intuitive but it is a well-known principal in acupuncture that the sharper and higher quality the needles the less painful the treatment as the needles pass more quickly through the area where the pain receptors are located allowing less time for the pain response to register.

Poor quality rollers often arrive with either blunt or bent needles which can make treatments very painful. The needle quality is the real technology behind the microneedle roller. The companies producing higher quality products spend their money on this and this is the reason to make sure you are comfortable with the supplier of the rollers you purchase.

The best quality rollers all use surgical stainless steel. This is the same quality of steel that is used in most modern surgical instruments. It has been shown to have the advantage of mechanical strength and lack of toxicity[1]. In recent years there has been a rise in the number of different materials being used to produce needles including the use of titanium. Despite the impressive sounding metal most people don't realise that these rollers often actually cost less to produce than the rollers which use higher quality stainless steel needles. In clinic I have seen no advantage in alternative metals and always use stainless steel.

The thickness of the needle is referred to as the gauge. The microneedles generally vary between 0.15 and 0.3 in gauge. Many companies make a lot of noise about the importance of their particular gauge to achieve best results. In clinic I prefer to use the larger gauges of 0.25 or 0.3 as I find this to be less painful. This sounds like a contradiction but I find that the thicker gauge is less likely to become blunt quickly and does not buckle under pressure. Blunt needles cause far more pain than the thicker gauge.

This becomes particularly important to people who are planning to reuse the roller at home as the thinner needles are likely to become blunt far more quickly and require more regular replacing. Interestingly a recent study has confirmed this theory showing that when using brand new sharp microneedles people cannot feel and difference in pain perception between microneedles of various width and thickness[2].

The ideal needle length for various treatments is discussed in a separate section later in the book.

Other Considerations

Finally always ensure any microneedle roller comes in tamper evident packaging and lists the method of sterilisation. Two common methods are gamma sterilisation and ethylene oxide symbolised by EO. Keep in mind that some cheaper rollers may list these methods and not carry them out. It is important to check. Some rollers are still hand assembled increasing the risk of needle stick injury in the factory. Make sure that any rollers you buy are machine assembled.

Chapter 2 - The History of Microneedling

Early Cosmetic Skin Needling in Ancient China

The first use of skin needling for cosmetic purposes was as part of the system of Chinese Medicine. The use of acupuncture needles for this purpose has existed for hundreds if not thousands of years.

More recently, in the 1970s, a professional group was formed by the Chinese government to investigate the effectiveness of cosmetic acupuncture as it is known. This group was disbanded in 1981 but left behind a legacy of techniques and protocols that are still in use today. In 1996 a collection of 300 cases of cosmetic acupuncture for facial rejuvenation performed in China reported that among 300 patients treated, 90% achieved marked results after one course of treatment[3].

Cosmetic acupuncture or acupuncture facial rejuvenation is of course very different to modern microneedling. The advent of the microneedle has changed the way most aesthetic skin needling is performed. There is however an important reason for looking at this history that is often overlooked.

In most cases where a treatment has existed in one form or another for such a long period you will usually find that the techniques have a much lower rate of side effects. Over an elongated period such as this clinicians have the chance to observe the effects of treatments over many generations. This makes it easier to observe any long term side effects. This is often very hard to do with a modern cosmetic treatment which is usually released to the public after only a few years of research.

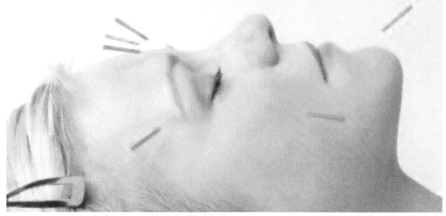

Image 3: Modern Cosmetic Acupuncture

The Development of Microneedling in the Western World
This is a more recent phenomenon based largely on technological advances in the methods of needle production. These advances have led to the development of the microneedle which has in turn allowed the development of the microneedle roller.

The first recorded use of microneedles in a scientific trial was in 1998. This trial was designed to demonstrate how microneedles could increase the absorption of products through the skin. They managed to demonstrate that microneedles of 0.15mm in length, left in the skin for 10 seconds resulted in an almost 10,000 fold increase in absorption of calcein by the skin after the microneedles were removed[4].

The use of microneedles to increase transdermal absorption has distinct advantages for those with impaired digestion as well as allowing clinicians to better target many drugs to reach the treatment area.

This research is on-going and several of the more recent findings are listed in the chapter on scientific research later in the book. This research has led to a variety of different delivery methods for drugs involving microneedles and has seen many advances in needle technology.

Most of these trials focus on stamps or plates to apply microneedling. It is the aesthetic industry that has seen the application of microneedle rollers, ascend to widespread popularity.

The Development of Collagen Induction Therapy
The first important report of the advantages of skin needling for cosmetic purposes in the west was by Orentreich and Orentreich in 1995[5]. The researchers cut below a depressed scar with a tri-bevelled hypodermic needle adjacent to the scar. They demonstrated that the introduction of a controlled trauma (such as a needle) initiates wound healing with consequent formation of connective tissue including increased collagen induction.

This is the first scientifically recorded evidence of what is often now referred to as 'collagen induction therapy'. Interestingly it is almost identical to an Ancient Chinese Medicine technique for treating scars called 'circling the dragon'. In this practice acupuncture needles are inserted below the scars from a number of directions with the intent purpose of improving the appearance of the scar. Although involving different terminology the techniques are almost identical.

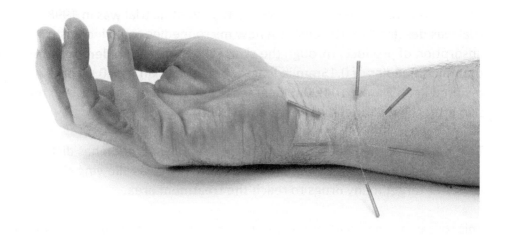

Image 4: Circling the Dragon: A Traditional Acupuncture Treatment for Scars

A year later in 1996 a plastic surgeon by the name of Dr Fernandes presented a paper to the International Society of Aesthetic Plastic Surgery (ISAPS) conference in Taiwan on the subject of microneedling[6]. This paper introduced a needle stamp he had developed to induce collagen production. This stamp was very similar to a Traditional Chinese Medicine device called the dermal hammer, 7 star needle or plum blossom needle which has been used for 100's of years for the treatments of scars and other cosmetic conditions. The principle difference was the advance in technology which allowed the production of shorter, thinner needles allowing these treatments to be performed far more easily and painlessly.

From this point onwards there was a great proliferation in scientific studies on cosmetic microneedling and its popularity grew rapidly.

There is some debate as to who actually invented the first modern microneedle roller. Many credit Dr Fernandes with inventing an early model containing 70 microneedles, while others claim it was invented in Germany. The truth behind this is hard to elicit but from the year 2000 onwards microneedle rollers grew rapidly in popularity and have become a mainstream cosmetic treatment across the Western world.

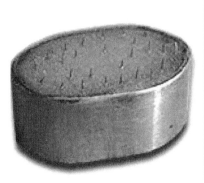 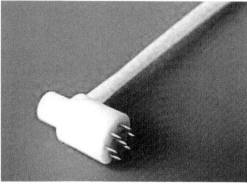

Image 5: A Comparison of Dr Fernandes Stamp with the Traditional 7 Star Needle

Chapter 3 - How Does it Work?

The microneedle roller works in two distinct ways. It increases transdermal absorption and it increases collagen induction. Each is best described separately.

A Refresher on the Anatomy of the Skin Influenced by Microneedling

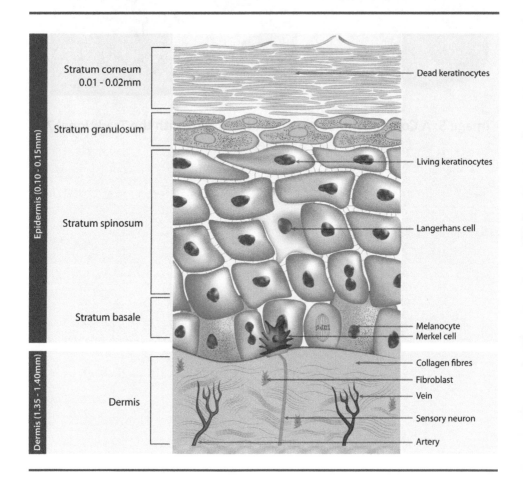

Diagram 1: Diagrammatic Representation of the Structures in the Skin

Stratum Corneum – This is the surface layer of the epidermis. It is a layer of flattened keratinocytes. It is this layer which provides the skins water proof barrier. As you can see it is only between 0.01-0.02mm thick so very short needles can be used to puncture it and increase transdermal absorption.

Stratum Granulosum – Consists of 3-5 layers of flattened keratinocytes undergoing cell death.

Stratum Spinosa – This is the second deepest layer of the epidermis. It consists of 8-10 layers of many sided keratinocytes. It is this layer in which dramatic thickening of the epidermis has been found following microneedle treatments.

Stratum Basale – This is the deepest layer of the epidermis. Some cells in this layer are stem cells which continually produce new keratinocytes. Stimulating and producing increased numbers of keratinocytes is an alternative explanation as to how microneedling produces results. If this is true much shorter needles can be used as this layer exists quite superficially as can be seen in the diagram.

Epidermis – This is composed of the 4 layers described above in thin skin which includes all skin except the palms and soles of the feet. It is generally believed that to induce collagen the needles must pass through this layer into the dermis to stimulate fibroblast activity. The epidermis is between 0.1 and 0.15mm thick. Due to the unevenness of skin a 0.5mm roller needle has been shown to be the shortest needle that consistently reaches the dermis to induce collagen.

Dermis – Lying below the epidermis the dermis comprises the majority of the thickness of the skin. Minor trauma to this area caused by the microneedles causes the fibroblasts to induce collagen as part of the wound healing process.

Keratinocyte – Make up 90% of cells in the epidermis and produce the protein keratin. Until recently they were little valued in cosmetic treatments and were often severely damaged in ablative treatments such as microdermabrasion while trying to reach the more commonly targeted fibroblasts in the dermis. Some clinicians are now rethinking this as the keratinocytes not only help thicken the epidermis but communicate with the fibroblasts which helps ensure healthy collagen production. Microneedling allows treatments to access the dermis and the fibroblasts directly with very little damage to the keratinocytes in the epidermis.

Fibroblast – Fibroblasts are cells located in the dermis which synthesize collagen. They have become something of a 'holy grail' to the cosmetic industry in recent decades as the production of collagen is a key goal in creating younger looking skin. As they are located in the dermis only needles of 0.5mm and longer can reach them directly.

Transdermal Absorption

Transdermal absorption is the absorption of products through the skin. As discussed previously the quantities of substances absorbed through the skin can be dramatically increased with the use of microneedling. Although often described in very complicated detail the way in which this is achieved is actually quite simple.

As the roller is passed over the skin the array of microneedles are inserted into the skin, piercing the stratum corneum and creating micro conduits or small channels for transport across the stratum corneum barrier. The needles are large enough to create micrometer-scale pathways through the skin for drug delivery of even the largest macromolecules. Once the substances have passed through the stratum corneum they diffuse through the highly permeable capillaries found in the superficial dermis and from there move into the main blood stream.

To put it very simply the needles create holes in the skin through which practically any substance can pass.

The stratum corneum is the outer barrier of the skin and is largely responsible for our skin being water proof. For decades scientists had worked on ways to improve the absorption of products through the skin. The development of a device that simply creates tiny holes in the outer layer of the skin appears to be the simplest and most effective way to do this. These holes rapidly close again restoring the barrier with very little recovery time.

Increased absorption of substances through the skin has several major advantages for the delivery of some pharmaceutical drugs. Firstly many patients do not absorb drugs taken orally due to impaired digestion often due to illness. This can mean the drug passes through the system without being absorbed and therefore without benefiting the patient. In other cases it is the drugs that are sensitive to the digestive environment of the patient. Some drugs are also more effective if they do not undergo the first pass effect of the liver during digestion. This first pass effect takes place when drugs are first absorbed through the digestive system. They then enter the hepatic portal system. As they pass through the liver the liver can metabolise many drugs before they have a chance to enter the systemic circulation.

The use of microneedling avoids many of the problems experienced through oral drug delivery. It does this without the inconvenience, pain and in many cases, fear of the hypodermic syringe.

It is worth noting here that although very small microneedles of 0.2 and 0.3mm can increase transdermal absorption at least one study has found that the 0.5mm needle length is the most effective at increasing this absorption[7]. Interestingly this study also found the 0.5mm needle length more effective for this purpose than the 1.5mm needles. It is believed this is because the 0.5mm roller delivers the substances to the ideal depth to allow maximum absorption by the minor capillaries.

One final point that it is important to make is that the most common side effect of microneedling treatments is dry skin. This is easy to understand when you realise that by puncturing the stratum corneum you are not only allowing an increase in absorption of products you also allow small amounts of the body's fluids to leak out. This is referred to as Trans-epidermal water loss (TEWL).

Collagen Induction Therapy
Unlike transdermal absorption, the process by which the microneedle rollers induct collagen, is extremely complicated and involves numerous biological substances. The basic principle however is easy to understand. The microneedles penetrate to the depth of the dermis where they create micro trauma. This micro trauma initiates the wound healing cascade. A wide variety of different cells are mobilised to the area in order to repair the wound. During this process new collagen is produced and old misaligned collagen is broken down. Over a period of months an entire new collagen and elastin matrix is laid down. This new matrix thickens the skin and improves the texture of the skin removing or reducing, a variety of wrinkles, scars and other cosmetic conditions.

Many people do not realise that in addition to creating new collagen, old collagen is broken down. In this way microneedling can actually assist in the treatment of scars and stretch marks. Simply inducing new collagen in these cases would not be effective. In fact an entirely new collagen and elastin matrix is formed. This effectively flattens out rough or uneven skin.

It is worth understanding that microneedling is not the only treatment that uses the wound healing cascade to produce new collagen. Ablative treatments such as microdermabrasion and chemical peels also use this method. The difference is that microneedling can produce this new collagen, elastin matrix without removing the epidermis. This results in far less trauma and does not damage the keratinocytes in the epidermis which play a role in the wound healing process.

For those who work in the field or who have a scientific background a more detailed summary is included below. The information I have just provided is how I usually explain the process to my clients most of whom do not have scientific training. For clinicians it is useful to remember this short explanation for this purpose. For home users it may be all the information you need and you may be happy to skip the next section.

Detailed Mechanism of Collagen Induction Therapy
Collagen induction therapy is dependent on the wound healing cascade. Wound healing is understood to occur in 3 phases. It is easier to describe each phase separately to avoid confusion. It is important to understand that all the phases and individual processes do not occur in a simple chronological order but in fact overlap.

Inflammatory Phase
As the microneedles penetrate through the epidermis to the dermis they rupture blood vessels causing the blood and serum to enter the surrounding tissues. Platelets in the blood then begin the clotting process. They also release chemotactic factors which attract further platelets as well as neutrophils and fibroblasts. The neutrophils then act to remove debris and kill bacteria in the area.

It is this stage of the wound healing process that has led many in the industry to insist that results can only be achieved with excessive bleeding of the skin. It is important to understand that even a smaller 0.5mm will produce a small amount of blood as the needles reach the level of the blood vessels. This small amount of blood vessel damage below the surface of the skin ensures adequate release of cytokines which ensure smooth healing. What has not been demonstrated but often assumed is that this process requires large quantities of blood seeping from the skin. Many clinicians are now finding that comparable results can be achieved without this excessive bleeding which will be discussed further later in the book.

As the platelets are exposed to collagen they release numerous cytokines including growth factors as well as pro-inflammatory factors. A number of these are of special importance for our purposes.

Fibrin and fibronectin cross link together to form a plug that prevents any further blood loss. This plug will remain the main structural support until collagen is deposited.

Some of these inflammatory factors increase vascular permeability allowing cells like neutrophils to pass through the vessel walls to the damaged area. This does not happen immediately. Straight after the injury the cell membranes release factors such as thromboxane's and prostaglandins that cause vasoconstriction to prevent further blood loss. The vasoconstriction lasts for between 5- 10 minutes. The vasodilation follows and peaks at about 20 minutes. This can be seen in gentle microneedling as the skin usually continues to become more flushed for up to 20 minutes. The main factor involved in causing vasodilation is histamine. Histamine is also largely responsible for the itchiness some patients experience after microneedling.

Some of the principal factors activated during this cascade are listed below.

Platelet derived growth factor (PDGF) attracts and promotes the proliferation of fibroblasts. This allows more collagen and elastin to be produced.

Transforming growth factor (TGF-b) attracts fibroblasts which migrate into the area after injury. They produce collagen type I and III. Collagen type III is the dominant form of collagen in the early stage of wound healing. They also produce elastin, glycosaminoglycans and proteoglycans and inhibit proteases that break down the intercellular matrix.

Fibroblast growth factors (FGF) promote an increase in fibroblasts, epidermal proliferation and new blood vessels.

Connective tissue activating peptide III promotes the production of the intercellular matrix. Restoring the matrix is vital because as discussed above partially breaking down the existing matrix contributes to the effectiveness of microneedling. Breaking down the old, uneven matrix and forming a new smoother version allow treatments to be effective against scars and stretch marks. The surge of activity this creates leads to the creation of more collagen and elastin.

During the inflammatory phase, macrophages begin to replace neutrophils from about 2 days after the injury. They continue to consume bacteria and damaged tissue. They also destroy the now decaying neutrophils. It is worth understanding that with microneedling there is very little connective tissue damage to be dealt with. Macrophages become particularly important from day 3 or 4 onwards as they release several growth factors including PDGF, FGF, TGF-b and Transforming Growth Factor (TGF-a) which stimulate the proliferation and migration of fibroblasts and the production of the extracellular matrix during the proliferative phase.

The migration of fibroblasts into the area usually begins 2-3 days after the injury and indicates the beginning of the proliferative phase even before the inflammatory phase has ended. The inflammatory phase usually lasts about 5 days after injury. Some clinicians are now focusing on elongating the inflammatory phase in the belief that this achieves better results. Unfortunately, elongating this phase also holds the potential to cause tissue damage and so is in my opinion best avoided[8].

Proliferative Phase
During the proliferative phase the keratinocytes located in the epidermis become one of the most important cells. Disruption of the basement membrane separating the epidermis from the dermis destroys the lamina lucida. This brings the basal keratinocytes into direct contact with the underlying collagen. This inactivates laminin and causes keratinocytes to change morphology and become mobile. They then migrate to cover the gap in the basement membrane.

This migration can begin as little as a few hours and is completed rapidly as the gaps created are so minimal. Once the keratinocytes have migrated across and joined together they start producing all the components to re-establish the basement membrane with laminin and collagens type IV and VII. Originally the keratinocytes begin migrating to close the gap without proliferating. Several days after the injury the keratinocytes begin to proliferate and start to thicken the epidermis particularly the stratum spinosa.

In the first 2-3 days after injury fibroblasts mainly migrate to the area and proliferate. It is only later that they become the main cells that lay down collagen matrix in the wound area. By the end of the first week fibroblasts are the main cells in the wound area.

Angiogenesis or neovascularisation occurs concurrently with fibroblast proliferation when endothelial cells migrate to the wound. Angiogenesis is vital for later stages of the wound healing process as the activity of fibroblasts and epithelial cells require oxygen and nutrients in order to function correctly. In the short term this low oxygen environment stimulates the fibroblasts to produce more TGF-b, PDGF and endothelial growth factor (EGF).

As explained above collagen type III is the main collagen in the early wound healing phase. The deposition peaks between 1 and 3 weeks after injury. This collagen combined with fibronectin remains the main substances providing tensile strength until the later stage of wound healing.

As fibroblasts are producing collagen, collagenases and other factors are simultaneously degrading it. During the first 2 stages of wound healing described the synthesis of collagen exceeds the destruction of it. The onset of the later maturation stage of wound healing is signalled by the return to balance of the creation and destruction of collagen.

Maturation and Remodelling
By the fifth day after injury the fibronectin matrix is laid down along the axis in which the fibroblasts are aligned. The collagen type III matrix is then laid down along this axis in the upper dermis just below the basal layer of the epidermis. Collagen type III is gradually replaced by collagen type I over a period of 6-12 months. As this phase progresses the tensile strength of the wound continues to increase.

It is important to realise that a single needle puncture would not produce significant results. However a microneedle roller containing 192 microneedles, produces more than 250 pricks in the skin per square cm when rolled across the area 15 times[9]. These tiny wounds placed so closely together produce a virtually constant sheet of new collagen just below the epidermis.

Keratinocytes an Alternative Target to Fibroblasts

Interestingly until recently it has been assumed that the target cells in microneedling were the fibroblasts to induce new collagen production. Dr Setterfield has recently advanced a theory that an alternative productive target may in fact be the keratinocyte[10]. Repeated micro injury to the keratinocytes releases anti fibrotic growth factors and improves communication between keratinocytes, melanocytes and fibroblasts. This assists fibroblasts to differentiate to form normal collagen and increased amounts of hyaluronic acid. This process not only forms new collagen but is ideal for wound healing.

This theory is important as the keratinocytes are located much closer to the skin surface in the epidermis. The fibroblasts are only located deeper in the skin at the level of the dermis. If the keratinocytes do play a larger role than previously thought it is very strong support for the use of much shorter needles. Longer needles may in fact not only be causing much greater tissue damage but may not in fact be enhancing results at all.

Chapter 4 - What Can Microneedling Benefit?

In this chapter we will examine which conditions microneedling is currently being used to assist. The current uses are far from exhaustive. It is my belief that as the mechanism of skin needling is better understood a wide variety of new therapeutic and cosmetic uses will enter common practice. Detailed procedures of how to treat each of the conditions listed below are included later in the book.

Facial Rejuvenation
This is of course a very general term which describes a variety of conditions. For our purposes these include wrinkles, sagging skin or skin laxity, UV damage and thinning skin.

Although all these conditions are of course different there are enough similarities in the causes and how they are treated to allow them to be explained together. I have avoided a long detailed explanation of the science behind the aging of the skin. There are numerous books written on the subject. For our purposes it is sufficient to say that loss of collagen and elastin in the skin is one of the main causes of loss of structural integrity in the skin over time.

These conditions can benefit from microneedling due to microneedling's ability to increase collagen induction, increase elastin and form a new collagen matrix which helps smooth out uneven skin, the most obvious example of which is wrinkles. The increase in elastin and collagen tightens skin to benefit and prevent sagging. Microneedling has also repeatedly been shown to thicken the skin so reducing the thinning of skin associated with aging.

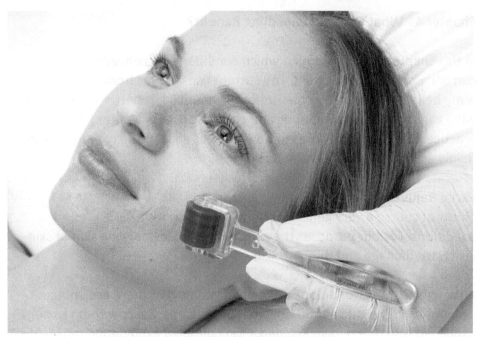
Image 6 – Facial Rejuvenation

Hand Rejuvenation
This technique is growing rapidly in popularity. It works in the same way as the facial rejuvenation treatments by stimulating collagen production and thickening the skin in the area.

Neck and Décolletage Rejuvenation
Again this is a recent technique that is growing rapidly in popularity. Microneedling has the ability to tighten loose skin around the neck and benefit aging and sun damaged skin across the décolletage through the induction of collagen in the area.

Sagging Upper Arms
Known colloquially as 'chicken wings', microneedling can help tighten the wrinkled skin produced by sagging in this area.

Scars
The treatment of scars is one of the most well documented uses of microneedling and has been partly responsible for its rapid growth in popularity.

Microneedling is beneficial on most types of scars with the exception of keloid scars. Keloid scars are usually identified by the fact that they grow beyond the original area of the wound.

Assuming that a scar is stable (so not a keloid) then microneedling can benefit both hypertrophic (raised scars) and atrophic scars (sunken scars) from a wide variety of causes including wounds, surgery and acne.

It is easy to understand how microneedling benefits scars. Scars are formed from collagen just like healthy skin. In healthy skin the collagen forms a basket weave pattern leaving the skin smooth. When scarring occurs the collagen fibres cross link and align principally in one direction. Under a microscope the fibres appear to run parallel to one another. Microneedling has the ability to break up old collagen bundles and help form a new collagen matrix in the form of the original basket weave of healthy skin.

Stretch Marks or Striae

Stretch marks result from rapid stretching of the skin associated with rapid growth. Both stretch marks and scars involve a misaligning of collagen fibres in the skin. Unlike scars stretch marks can only form when there is no longer a good support structure available in the surrounding tissue. For a stretch mark to form the underlying structure must already be compromised. This makes stretch marks more difficult to treat than scars.

Having said this microneedling can be of great benefit for stretch marks. It works in a similar way to the treatment of scarring. It breaks down the old misaligned collagen bundles and forms a new matrix in the area. The underlying weakness of the tissues means that results often take longer to produce but can be impressive when they are achieved.

Cellulite

Cellulite at a basic level is caused by fat cells becoming swollen and pushing through the collagen and elastin matrix. When the collagen and elastin matrix is healthy it has a basket weave formation producing smooth skin. When the fat cells begin to push through and distort this matrix it produces the dimple like appearance associated with cellulite.

Many clinics now use microneedling to affectively assist this condition. The exact mechanism by which this works is not yet understood. It is possible that microneedling benefits this condition by producing a new stronger collagen and elastin matrix which can then better control the swollen fat cells.

It will be interesting to see if this idea is confirmed by future research as the cause of microneedling's effectiveness in this condition.

Hyperpigmentation

The causes of hyperpigmentation are complicated as are the ways in which microneedling benefits it. Many cases are found in individuals with darker skin such as those of Africa and southern India origins. Excessive sun exposure is a key cause but there can be a variety of other causes including acne vulgaris or other skin injuries.

Scientifically the main cause of hyperpigmentation is disorders of the melanocytes which produce melanin. The mechanism by which microneedling benefits hyperpigmentation has not been studied but it may be that it is due to microneedling's ability to help normalise the signalling between keratinocytes and melanocytes and normalise melanogenesis and melanocyte differentiation.

Clinically I have seen good results with many cases of hyperpigmentation but it is by no means guaranteed and it is often hard to determine exactly which patients will benefit most. Where an underlying autoimmune disease such as Addison's or Cushing's disease is present the skin should not be treated as the treatment is unlikely to achieve results.

It is important to note that microneedling is considered a very safe treatment that can be applied to individuals with darker southern Indian or African skin. Unlike treatments such as microdermabrasion it has not been linked to any loss of pigmentation with repeated treatments.

Age Spots

Microneedling can benefit small changes in pigmentation caused by age. It is likely that it does this through the same mechanism by which it assists hyperpigmentation.

Rosacea

Rosacea is of course a chronic skin condition characterised by redness of the face. The use of microneedling to benefit rosacea is relatively recent but has shown positive early results.

Medically rosacea is associated with a hypersensitivity of the blood vessels in the face. The constant expansion of these blood vessels causes the redness of the face. This constant expansion leads to weakening of the collagen and connective tissue between the blood vessels. Once this is damaged the blood vessels can expand more easily and are closer to the surface making the appearance of rosacea worse. Long term rosacea also leads to scar tissue forming in the skin.

Microneedling benefits this condition by increasing the collagen induction in the area and strengthening the connective tissue so reducing the blood vessels expansion. This can dramatically reduce or even remove the redness. Microneedling's ability to benefit scars is also useful to those who suffer from chronic rosacea.

Rosacea is often associated with certain trigger factors such as sunlight, foods, beverages, temperature changes and medications. This makes it hard to ever claim a cure for rosacea as it has a habit of recurring when a patient is exposed to their particular trigger factors. Having said this microneedling can produce good results in reducing the redness and improving the appearance of rosacea. It also reduce the frequency and severity of attacks.

It is important to note that microneedling can be used on most cases of rosacea but should not be used on nodular or pustular rosacea. These conditions can be treated once the outbreak has cleared.

Acne

The use of microneedling on acne is highly effective but also difficult to perform effectively. Microneedling can be used to increase the circulation in the area and deliver a range of substances more directly into the skin that benefit the acne.

Unfortunately rolling across active acne will spread the bacteria. This means that treatments must be performed in between outbreaks or around active areas.

What makes this so important to understand is that many people who wish to treat acne scarring are still suffering from outbreaks of acne. In this case you must build up slowly, working around the acne until it can be improved enough to perform full treatments.

If you are planning to treat acne with microneedling it is important to remember that many acne medications are contraindicated with microneedling and it is worth reading about which medications to avoid later in the book before proceeding.

Enlarged Pores
Enlarged pores are particularly common on the nose but can be found elsewhere on the face. Traditionally in China they were treated by tapping the area with a seven star needle (pictured earlier) to increase the circulation in the area. Over time this reduced the size of the pores.

In modern clinics the microneedle roller can be used to serve the same purpose in a more convenient way. It improves the texture of the skin by inducting collagen in the area and so reduces the size and adverse appearance of the enlarged pores.

Hair Loss
Microneedling can effectively benefit several different types of hair loss. The first of these is Androgenetic Alopecia, more commonly known as male pattern baldness. Despite its more common name it also occurs in women in the form of thinning hair. This is the most common form of hair loss and also the type microneedling is most effective at assisting.

Microneedling is also effective in assisting postpartum hair loss. Although this type of hair loss naturally resolves over time, microneedling appears to reduce the amount of hair lost and speed up the recovery time.

Many microneedling clinics are also using microneedling to treat Alopecia Areata which involves loosing small circles of hair and is usually associated with an autoimmune disorder or response. Clinically I am far more reluctant to treat this type of hair loss as there are often complicating factors.

Microneedling assists hair loss by increasing the release of endothelial growth factor which has been shown to promote hair growth, increase follicle and hair size and benefit Platelet derived growth factor which assists the interactions that lead to hair canal formation[11,12].

In practice the products used with the microneedling roller also play a large role in the effectiveness of hair loss treatments. Many large clinics around the world now use the rollers with products such a minoxidil. An alternate I use in clinic are traditional Chinese herbal formulas used to promote hair growth. Most of these herbs have been used for thousands of years for these purposes and many of the therapeutic claims of these herbs are now being validated by scientific research. This includes herbs such as ginseng which are now being researched to treat hair loss and are showing very promising results[13]. These have reduced risks of side effects and often greater patient compliance due to the dramatically reduced costs compared to minoxidil.

Chapter 5 - The Research behind Microneedling

Transdermal Absorption Research

Increasing transdermal absorption of a variety of substances is an on-going goal of both cosmetic and therapeutic research. The principal aim is to allow greater quantities of therapeutic drugs or cosmetic applications to pass through the strateum corneum and so enter the systematic circulation without having to pass through the digestion and the first pass effect of the liver.

Various other methods have and continue to be explored with this aim. These include enhanced absorption through the applications of chemicals (14,15,16); and the application of various other physical methods such as iontophoresis (17); sonophoresis [18,19]; and electroporation [20,21].

In comparison to these methods microneedling provides a very safe, painless and effective method of increasing transdermal absorption. This summary of the research is far from conclusive as there is now such a large body of evidence on this subject. I have instead selected a range of the more important studies which provide a good insight into why researchers are so excited about the potential of microneedling to increase transdermal absorption.

The first major study of microneedles to increase transdermal absorption was carried out in 1998. This study found that microneedles of 0.15mm in length applied for 10 seconds could increase the absorption of the drug calcein by almost 10,000 times compared to applying the drug to the skin without the microneedles[4].

In 2002 a study by Matriano et al. used micro-projections of 0.33mm in length to deliver a vaccine[22]. He found the immune response to be 50 times greater than that observed after the same dose was delivered by a hypodermic syringe intramuscularly or subcutaneously. Since then a lot of research has focused on using microneedles to deliver vaccines. A 2009 review of the evidence concluded that for a variety of vaccines microneedles will be more effective, less painful, safer and more dose sparing than the current application of either subcutaneous or intramuscular injections[23].

It is interesting to note that it is well documented that the ancient Chinese practiced a form of vaccination called variolation by scratching the skin to immunise against small pox[24]. This technique of variolation was later improved in Europe by Edward Jenner using cow pox. He then coined the term vaccination. The important point is that these early vaccination methods were conducted at the surface of the skin, the same depth at which microneedling is showing such promising results.

A 2004 study showed a 90% increase in the absorption of the drug desmopressin when using a 0.2mm microneedle[25]. This was very impressive as desmopressin does not normally absorb through the skin at all without the use of microneedles. This shows that microneedling can not only increase the absorption of drugs through the skin but it can allow substances that could not normally cross the skin to penetrate. This becomes important for our understanding later in the book.

As a final example of just how effective microneedling can be a 2003 paper described, that based on current results a 1cm square patch applied with a standard concentration of insulin is enough to meet the daily needs of most diabetics[26].

The above studies were conducted using a variety of needle stamps, rollers and other devices to insert microneedles. The results are still very relevant as the needle length and penetration are similar or identical in most cases.

The exact amount of a substance absorbed through the skin with the use of microneedles is dependent on a number of factors including the size of the drug molecule, how quickly the drugs breaks down, whether the drug is applied before or after needling, the diameter and length of the needles, the spaces between the needles and the method of insertion. There have been many recent studies that demonstrate that the microneedle rollers have an effective distribution of needles to dramatically increase transdermal absorption[7,27,28].

The current difficulty in determining the exact dose of a substance delivered during microneedling is presenting difficulties in convincing regulators that microneedling is a more useful method of drug delivery than hypodermic or oral delivery. If this is overcome we will almost certainly see microneedling patches or rollers as a common method of delivering pharmaceutical drugs in future.

It is clear from these studies that microneedles used correctly can dramatically increase absorption of a wide variety of substances through the skin. It has also been demonstrated that microneedling can allow drugs that would otherwise be unable to do so, to cross the barrier of the skin.

This fact has not been lost on the cosmetic industry which has dramatically embraced this research as part of the growing body of evidence supporting the effectiveness of microneedle rollers.

Collagen Induction Research
The research on transdermal absorption has largely focused on medical applications and has therefore used a variety of microneedling devices. The research on collagen induction has on the other hand focused almost exclusively on the microneedle rollers to achieve aesthetic results. Below is a short summary of some of the main studies demonstrating how effective the rollers can be for a variety of conditions.

The earliest major study examining the effects of collagen induction therapy was carried out in 2006[29]. Biopsies were taken from various parts of the body of 10 patients who had been treated once with a microneedle roller. Six to eight weeks later, another biopsy was taken from the needled skin. New collagen and elastin fibre formation was obvious and quite dramatic. On average, an increase of new fibres of 206% was observed and in one case a 1,000% increase was recorded. There was an absence of any signs of overt tissue damage. Interestingly although this study used a 1.5mm roller new collagen was only found to a depth of 0.5-0.6mm. This supports the principle of using shorter needles discussed later in the book.

Another larger study followed in 2008 [30]. This was a retrospective analysis of 480 patients with fine wrinkles, lax skin, scarring, and stretch marks treated with percutaneous collagen induction. On average, patients rated their improvement between 60 and 80 per cent better than before the treatment. Histologic examination was carried out in 20 patients and showed a considerable increase in collagen and elastin deposition at 6 months postoperatively. The epidermis demonstrated 40 per cent thickening of the stratum spinosa. Again this increase was located very shallowly in the second deepest layer of the epidermis.

A 2010 in vivo study further supported this evidence and provided more insights into the mechanism[31]. The study demonstrated a 140% increase in epidermal thickness and an increase in gene and protein expression of collagen 1, and growth factors such as VEGF and EGF. It also demonstrated an increase in the number of and thickness of the collagen bundles.

For those concerned with the risk of hyper pigmentation with cosmetic treatments a 2008 study showed that skin needling did not result in any loss of melanocytes[32]. The authors conclusion was that microneedling improved the skins appearance and quality without the risk of dyspigmentation.

Several studies have dealt specifically with the use of microneedling to reduce scars. In 2009 a trial of 37 people showed 34 of them receiving an improvement of 1 or 2 grades in the appearance of the scars after treatment with a microneedle roller[33].

This research was followed by a 2010 trial which showed that 16 patients suffering post burn scars treated with a microneedle roller rated their improvement at an average of 80%[34]. Histological examination 12 months later showed considerable increases in collagen and elastin and a 45% thickening of the stratum spinosa.

Applying the principals used to treat scarring a preliminary study of 22 women suffering stretch marks showed significant increase in collagen and elastin fibres in the area 6 months after treatment[35].

In 2010 a very small initial evaluation of the application of microneedling to hand rejuvenation was carried out[36]. This has become a popular technique and the study showed a visual improvement in both skin texture and skin tightening.

A 2011 study directly compared microneedling to Intense Pulsed Light (IPL) therapy. The study concluded that microneedling resulted in greater skin thickening and expression of collagen type 1 as well as total collagen content[37].

A 2010 study has provided support to the idea of microneedling improving hair loss. This study used a microneedle roller in conjunction with L-ascorbic acid[38]. The results showed an increase in hair growth with this method. Whether it was due to the microneedling alone or the combination of treatments remains to be explored.

Chapter 6 – Comparing Microneedling to Conventional Cosmetic Treatments

We have seen clear evidence that microneedling works but it is certainly not the only cosmetic treatment available. In this chapter I will explain some of the advantages of microneedling over many conventional cosmetic treatments. It is also important to discuss potential interactions with many of these popular treatments.

Ablative Treatments

Medically ablation refers to the surgical removal of a part of the body. Ablative cosmetic treatments are understood as those which remove or severely damage the outer layer of skin. The level of damage caused varies between treatments. In most cases it involves the removal of one or several layers of the epidermis.

Microneedling and ablative treatments have a common goal. Both treatments aim to cause some level of trauma in the dermis level of the skin. In so doing they stimulate fibroblast activity directly so increasing collagen production. Although both microneedling and ablative treatments both use the trauma in the dermis to initiate the wound healing cascade and induce collagen there is a large difference in the mechanism they use to achieve this.

Ablative treatments either remove or in some cases damage the epidermis which can lead to scar tissue. Microneedling in comparison leaves the epidermis intact as the needle punctures created disappear in a matter of hours.

By removing the external layer of the skin ablative treatments increase recovery times, infection risk, dehydration and the potential for dyspigmentation. They also severely damage or even remove the keratinocytes located in the epidermis which are known to influence the regulation of collagen production.

Prior to the advent of the microneedle roller ablative treatments were considered the most effective way to influence collagen production in the dermis. Microneedling produces all the advantages of ablative treatments without the risks and discomfort associated with damaging or removing the epidermis.

Possibly the best known ablative treatments are microdermabrasion, chemical peels and laser resurfacing. Each works in a slightly different way and is best discussed individually

Microdermabrasion

Microdermabrasion is also referred to as mechanical exfoliation, skin resurfacing or micro-resurfacing. There are a number of different methods but they all involve removing varying levels of the outer layers of skin. Most use some form or abrasive particles that are passed across the skin at high speed removing the outer layer. The level of skin removed in microdermabrasion is dependent on the clinician's judgement. Many only remove superficial levels of the stratum corneum while others will remove deeper layers of skin. By removing the outer layers of skin microdermabrasion stimulates fibroblast activity which leads to collagen induction. In addition to this, by removing the outer layers of the skin, microdermabrasion can increase the absorption of products through the skin.

By removing the outer layers of skin microdermabrasion creates much greater risk of colour changes in the skin, loss of pigmentation, UV sensitivity weeping skin and skin infections as the skin is without its natural barrier to the outside world. The issue of pigmentation loss has been quite well documented recently. This has led many people with darker skin to seek alternative treatments such as microneedling. In addition microdermabrasion can involve much longer recovery times and is not suitable for those with compromised immune systems or suffering diabetes. In contrast microneedling can be used with both groups with due consideration to the severity of the condition.

When microneedling was first introduced many exponents recommended that it be used in conjunction with microdermabrasion. This practice is no longer common as it has proven to be unnecessary. Both treatments used alone can very successfully stimulate collagen production and using them together is more likely to increase pain, incur side effects and affect recovery times.

If considering using the two treatments in conjunction I recommend waiting until the skin has completely healed from the microdermabrasion before beginning a series of microneedling treatments. This can take between 2-8 weeks depending on the severity of the inflammation.

Chemical Peels

Chemical peels use a wide variety of chemicals producing varying degrees of severity of reaction. This makes it hard to generalise.

Different peels are designed to remove different levels of the skin. Peels that remove the largest amount of skin are associated with the greatest risk. Side effects of deeper peels include pigmentation changes, skin atrophy and textural changes.

The deepest peels such as traditional phenol peels required general anaesthetic due to the severe pain involved. More modern chemical peels can be performed with lower levels of anaesthetic.

The advantages of microneedling over chemical peels are similar to those for microdermabrasion. If using the two treatments in conjunction ensure all signs of inflammation from the peel have cleared before performing microneedling.

Laser Skin Resurfacing (LSR)

LSR is the use of either a carbon dioxide (CO_2) or Er:yag laser which are 2 different laser wavelengths. The lasers wound the skin to the dermis level. The healing process then employs the fibroblasts to induce collagen.

Unlike the two previous ablative treatments it does not actually remove the outer layers of the skin. It is considered ablative because of the thermal damage it often causes to the epidermal layers it must pass through to reach the dermis. When using a CO_2 laser for example the water in the tissues absorbs the laser often causing the temperature of the water to rise to more than 100°C. Thermal damage caused by laser resurfacing results in scar tissue in the area treated and increased risks of hypopigmentation. As the epidermis is damaged, the patient may experience oozing from the skin for around 2 weeks with the redness often persisting for 12 weeks of more.

This treatment has become increasingly popular as it has lower risks of infection than microdermabrasion and permits the surgeon greater control in varying the depth to which the skin is wounded. Microneedling has an obvious advantage in its ability to influence collagen production without risking scarring. The other major advantages of microneedling over LSR is the not insignificant cost difference with laser machines often costing tens of thousands of dollars which clinicians have to recoup in treatment fees. The performance and safety of lasers is also often largely dependent on the training and skill of the clinician with risks being increased where this training is inadequate.

Non Ablative Treatments
These treatments do not remove the outer layer of the skin and have the advantage of leaving the epidermis intact. Microneedling falls into this category. The advantage of leaving the surface layer of the skin intact is faster recovery times and less potential side effects.

Botulinum Toxin
Botulinum is a protein produced by bacteria. It is considered the most powerful neurotoxin ever discovered. Its use is widespread in the cosmetic industry under brand names like Botox, Dysport and Xeomin.

Botulinum toxin works by simply blocking the transfer of signals from the nerves to the muscles (neuromuscular transmission). The patient then simply cannot contract the muscle concerned almost instantly removing many wrinkles and altering the faces appearance. Microneedling in comparison stimulates the body's own natural wound healing response so producing the body's own collagen to create results. This takes more time but produces more natural and longer lasting results.

It is worth noting that once patients start Botulinum toxin it is very difficult to stop as the results wear off rapidly and are very noticeable to friends and family as they do so. Microneedling in comparison can be done in a series of treatments to produce long lasting results without a dramatic reduction in effect in the future.

The difference in potential health concerns must also be addressed. As part of my definition of holistic microneedling I stipulated that treatments must not in any way jeopardise health. The debate on the long term effects of Botulinum toxin still rages. Currently no long term side effects have been determined though this has not stopped the FDA producing a recent warning about a brand of Botulinum toxin after several deaths[39]. Patients and students often ask when it is safe to perform microneedling after Botulinum toxin. The answer to this is that there has been no research into this subject despite some clinics using the treatments together for many years.

In clinic I always wait between 2- 4 weeks after an injection before performing microneedling. This allows a very safe margin of error in case there is any underlying inflammation or bruising from the injections.

I also warn the clients that there is a chance the microneedling may reduce the length of time that the effects of botulinum toxin last. I believe this is highly probable as microneedling dramatically increases the body's natural healing processes and also dramatically increases the blood flow in the area. This can flush an area of skin and potentially remove any substances identified as foreign by the body. It is highly likely that this process may speed up the removal of the botulinum toxin and speed up the recovery from what the body considers a foreign invasion. My results in clinic seem to support this idea.

Microneedling can also provide an excellent way for patients who have been using botulinum toxin for some time to stop on-going injections if they so choose. It does this by starting to induct collagen before the botulinum toxin wears off. By doing this the sudden increase in lines associated with the botulinum toxin wearing off is not as noticeable. I usually recommend starting treatment at least 3 months before the botulinum toxin usually wears off to achieve results in these cases.

Dermal Fillers
Dermal fillers are injectable products designed to correct wrinkles and other depressions in the skin. The most common forms of dermal fillers in use at present are those based on hyaluronic acid. Previously collagen injections of both bovine and human engineered collagen were more common but these have gradually been withdrawn from the market in most countries.

Hyaluronic acid is the most prominent glycosaminoglycan in the skin. The most well-known brand of Hyaluronic acid is probably Restylane which is produced by fermentation in bacterial cultures of equine streptococci. It is believed to be chemically identical to the hyaluronic acid produced by humans in the skin.

As hyaluronic acid is not as readily identified as a foreign material by the body's immune system, microneedling should not increase its elimination in the way I believe it does with botulinum toxin. I have to some extent found this to be the case in clinic though more evidence would be needed to draw any conclusions.

As in the case of the Botulinum toxin microneedling has the advantage of working with the body's natural healing system and can produce longer lasting and more natural looking results than dermal fillers.

As with all other treatments, I suggest waiting until any sign of inflammation from the injections have been eliminated before performing microneedling. It is also worth remembering that hyaluronic acid has a heparin like effect that increases the rate of bruising. For this reason it is better to avoid performing the 2 treatments simultaneously to avoid excess bruising.

IPL – Intense Pulsed Light
IPL has become very popular in recent years as an alternative to laser resurfacing. Unlike laser resurfacing it is non-ablative so producing shorter recovery times and less post-procedural changes. IPL devices contain a non-coherent filtered flash lamp that emits a broad wavelength spectrum of 560nm to 1200nm, delivering a high peak in short pulses.
IPL has been shown to increase collagen type 1 and type 3 so can potentially produce similar results to microneedling[40,41].

Interestingly IPL is one of the few therapies where a scientific comparison with microneedling has been undertaken. Although only a preliminary study it demonstrated that after 3 weeks of treatment microneedling increased expressions of type 1 and total collagen significantly more so than IPL[37]. In addition microneedling also produced greater thickening of the skin than IPL.

Microneedling also appears to have several other advantages over IPL. These include the lower cost of the rollers compared to pulsed light machines, the ease of use and the increased public perception of risks associated with laser and light treatments particularly amongst those interested in natural treatments.

Part 2 – The Holistic Approach to Microneedling

Overview

Holistic microneedling involves combining the best of the modern scientific developments with a holistic paradigm that allows us to achieve greater results with fewer side effects.

Microneedling is unusual amongst cosmetic treatments. It can draw upon a long history of the safe effective skin needling in the form of acupuncture usage over thousands of years. Yet it also has a strong scientific principle and a rapidly growing body of scientific evidence demonstrating its results. In addition, it works by producing the body's own natural collagen. It does this in a way that causes no lasting damage and does not need to involve the addition of synthetic or potentially toxic chemicals. It also avoids the unknowns of the wide variety of light and laser therapies rapidly being released onto the market.

Microneedling is non-surgical and involves very short and gentle recovery times. More than any other cosmetic treatment microneedling naturally lends itself to being a breakthrough in the field of holistic therapies. Why then has no one even considered the idea of applying microneedling holistically until now?

I believe the answer to this lies in the underlying philosophy of the cosmetic industry. The initial developers of modern microneedling were largely surgeons. They developed the treatments in accordance with their current practices. Hence the earliest use of micro needle rollers were performed in a surgical environment, under general anaesthetic with a 3.0mm needle length roller (the skin only has an average thickness of 1.5mm). Under these conditions the wound healing process was extensive and very draining on the body so topical and often internal vitamin supplementation was required. Anaesthesia was a large issue as the needles were penetrating through the skin to the subcutaneous layer.

These initial pioneers set the stage for what became known as medical skin needling across Europe and later the rest of the Western world. This early model of microneedling use was clearly unsustainable. The costs of a hospital setting and general anaesthetic put the treatments out of the reach of most. As more research has been done it has gradually found that the same or in some cases even better results can actually be achieved with shorter needles. This has allowed microneedling to spread to less formidable surroundings such as beauty salons and ultimately the home use market. As these practices changed very few ever questioned the continuing need for the high dose vitamins or anaesthetics or excessively long needles.

Nearly all companies in the market today have simply adopted unquestioningly the original practices which were designed for microneedling in a hospital setting. Even the new home use roller companies attempt to duplicate these practices with cheap vitamin and mineral creams. As a marketing gimmick a company will occasionally add a minute dose of an herbal or natural supplement to the usual vitamin creams but overall the idea of actually performing holistic microneedling treatments has remained unknown in the industry.

In the following chapters I will outline the 3 principles of holistic microneedling, why they work and how to apply them.

Principle 1 – Use Only Natural Substances during Microneedling Treatments

Chapter 7 - Why Use Natural Products?

A Review of Transdermal Absorption and the Potential Issues

Earlier we examined the increase in transdermal absorption caused by microneedling. This ability to increase transdermal absorption has been capitalised upon by the cosmetic industry. Practically any pharmaceutical drug or vitamin compound that has been shown to have significant anti aging properties can now be applied with the microneedle roller and absorbed in far greater quantities. In some cases drugs or substances that previously could not cross the skin barrier at all can now enter the blood stream with the aid of microneedling[25].

The great potential benefit of this increase has allowed most in the industry to ignore any potential down side. For some time I have had some reservations about this. As discussed above substances that are absorbed through the skin with microneedling enter the small dermis capillaries virtually unaltered. If these same substances had been taken orally they would have gone through the digestive system. Anything that is in the digestive tract is still medically considered to be outside the body until it has managed to penetrate through the walls of the stomach or intestines. Amongst other things these walls and the substances they secrete are designed to break down some compounds that would be harmful to us if allowed to enter the blood stream directly.

By using substances with the microneedle roller we are in fact bypassing the body's first layer of defence and allowing them to enter systemic circulation in far higher quantities than would have previously been possible. This is very useful if the products applied are medicinal and non-toxic but disastrous if they are toxic.

It should be pointed out that this is an issue not just for products used during the treatment but also for products used at home before or after the treatment. Some products used on the skin earlier in the day can remain there for hours. Many sunburn creams are a good example of this as are most forms of make-up and many moisturisers. If the face is not cleansed thoroughly before the treatment any substances still on the skin may be absorbed in much greater quantities. This can be a particular concern for people who treat themselves at home who may not cleanse the face as thoroughly as in a clinical environment. In fact many companies that sell rollers for home use do not even mention this in their literature so users are not even aware of any risk.

There is also an on-going debate as to how long the micro channels created remain open. Some studies indicate that the micro channels were undetectable in just 20-30 minutes under a light microscope[42]. In contrast another study found that the electrical resistance of the skin remained significantly less for up to 30 hours indicating that transdermal absorption may remain increased during this time[43].

Any substances applied during this time following a microneedling treatment may be absorbed in higher quantities than normal and other substances that would not normally be absorbed at all can often enter the bloodstream. Any products applied to the skin during this time with potentially toxic ingredients should of course be avoided but very few companies warn users about this.

Occasionally the literature suggests avoidance of other products afterwards due to the increased risk of infection. The risk of infection is actually very low. There is rarely a mention of any potential risks with the increased absorption, only the benefits.

There is no fool proof solution for ensuring that only beneficial products are applied to the skin after treatment. This is particularly difficult for clinicians as we do not have full control of our client's behaviour after they leave the clinic. There is also no definitive list of products or chemicals that should be avoided. There are simply too wide a variety of chemicals in the personal products we now use to research them all in conjunction with microneedling. This creates something of a guessing game.

As the micro channels through the skin gradually close over time the highest risk is during and directly after treatment. To minimise this I usually ask clients to avoid applying anything to the skin after microneedling other than what I have provided them with. The products I use are all natural and will be discussed later. I prefer where possible to perform microneedling treatments in the afternoon and evenings as clients are less likely to have a social engagement. They can then wait until the following morning to apply make-up and other products. For those using microneedle rollers at home the advice is the same. Try to perform the treatments at night at home and avoid the application of make-up, moisturisers, shampoos or other skin products until at least the next morning.

Given the higher potential for toxicity and the relative unknown of how a variety of substances will react when absorbed trans dermally in higher doses it is best to opt for the most natural products possible that can still achieve the desired results. In most cases there are is a variety of products that can produce just as good if not better results without the potential risks or side effects of many synthetic products.

Products Currently Used with Microneedling in the Cosmetic Industry?
Currently a wide variety of substances for both topical and oral application are often prescribed during a course of microneedling. Interestingly these products vary at least slightly from company to company but many companies still claim that results will not be achieved without the application of their particular products.

Although there is quite a range of common products for topical application, the most common ones are Vitamin A in a variety of forms, Vitamin C and E, Alpha Lipoic, Omega 3, Glutathione, Colostrum, Resveratrol and Copper Peptides. Many groups now provide a unique branded combination of these and other products in a cream form combined with preservatives, stabilisers and fillers.

There is currently no evidence that microneedling works better in combination with these products. In fact several of the most impressive results were in fact achieved by 'dry needling' or the use of no products with the microneedling treatments[29,33]. By this I am not suggesting that there are not products that can enhance the results of microneedling or reduce the side effects. I simply want to point out that a lot of industry advertising suggests that their products are inseparable from achieving results with microneedling. The evidence shows this is not the case.

The rationale for the use of the above products in combination with microneedling is largely derived from the wound healing process. Wounds require certain vitamins, minerals and other compounds in order to heal effectively. These vitamins and minerals are produced naturally by a healthy person allowing healing every time we injure ourselves. By supplying these nutrients topically in large doses it is believed that they will heal more quickly and effectively. As discussed there is currently no evidence to show that this is necessary with microneedling and several examples that it probably is not.

Special note should also be made of the use of Vitamin A topically in a variety of different forms. Vitamin A has proven anti aging benefits when used alone topically and so was a natural candidate for the cosmetic industry to combine with microneedling. Unfortunately Vitamin A is also well known to produce redness, dryness and often flaky skin after use. Dryness and redness are also the most common complaint following a microneedling treatment as the epidermis is pierced and water is lost through the holes in this barrier. When microneedling and vitamin A are combined far more severe redness, dryness and flaky skin is experienced by the user for longer periods of time.

Additionally like oral consumption of Vitamin A, topical use can also be a cause of Hypervitaminosis A Syndrome[44]. This occurs when the liver's maximum stores of vitamin A are exceeded and the vitamin A enters the circulation causing systemic toxicity. Europeans have known about Hypervitaminosis A since 1597 when cases were recorded from eating polar bear liver which is particularly high in vitamin A (The traditional culture of the Inuit of course already knew about this and did not eat it!)[45].

The risk is very small and cases from topical application are rare but it must be considered that the risks are increased when used in conjunction with microneedling which increases transdermal absorption.

It is also important to understand that Vitamin A is not one homogenous substance. It describes a myriad of retinoid products and more are being developed all the time. This incorporates another unknown into the equation.

One of the principles of holistic microneedling is to achieve the maximum results with the absolute minimum risk. Given that the use of vitamin A has not been demonstrated to improve treatment results and the potential negative side effects it can produce I believe Vitamin A is unnecessary for use in microneedling treatments.

In addition to the vitamins and minerals mentioned above several companies are now combining microneedling with epidermal growth factor (EGF). EGF has the benefit of increasing cell division so can be useful for wound and burn healing. Unfortunately by increasing cell division it can also increase tumour growth[46]. The largest risk is if EGF is taken internally. The results of repeated use on unbroken skin are currently unknown and there is concern that it may lead skin cells to over produce. Psoriasis is a common example of skin cells over producing. When used with microneedling which increases transdermal absorption it must be considered that the risks mentioned above are magnified. For this reason I would highly recommend against the use of any products containing a genuine dose of EGF with microneedling.

Are Synthetic Vitamins Natural?
This is a popular notion that warrants discussion. The vast majority of vitamins produced in topical creams are usually produced synthetically in a laboratory and yet are often advertised as natural as they are reputed to be identical to vitamins that occur naturally in plant and animal sources. This is not always the case.

Until the 1950's it was believed that synthetically produced vitamin E was identical to the natural occurring form. As science advanced and the ability to determine more accurately the chemical structure of vitamins improved this was dramatically disproved[47,48]. Trials have now shown that naturally occurring Vitamin E is 50% more bioavailable than synthetically produced Vitamin E[48].

As our understanding of chemistry and biology continues to grow, we may find other apparently identical synthetic vitamins are actually identified by the body as 'unnatural' and absorbed in different ways. Unfortunately until that research evolves synthetic vitamins will continue to be advertised and sold as 'natural products' and assumed rather than known to be identical to their naturally occurring forms.

It is interesting at this point to examine how synthetic vitamins are produced. A common production method for a vitamin A compound is a good place to start. This method is used to produce the commonly used form of retinyl palmitate which is one of the less irritant forms of the Vitamin A compounds used.

A Description of Vitamin A Palmitate Production[49]

1.   Vitamin A acetate is prepared synthetically by treatment of pseudoionone with sulphuric acid, and by condensation of the resulting β-ionone with methyl chloroacetate to the "glycidic ester" intermediate, which is decarboxylated to β-C14-aldehyde.
2.   Grignard reaction of β-C14-aldehyde with 3-methyl-2-penten-4-yn-1-ol gives the C20-alkynediol, which is catalytically hydrogenated to C20-alkenediol.
3.   Reaction of C20-alkenediol with acetic anhydride and subsequent dehydration with hydrobromic acid gives then vitamin A acetate. The resulting crude product is purified by crystallization from methanol, dried, and then filled into containers.
4.   Vitamin A acetate reacts with methyl palmitate in the presence of sodium methoxide (or alternatively sodium hydroxide) in a suitable solvent to give Vitamin A Palmitate, which is isolated by extraction. The product is isolated by vacuum-concentration and then filled into containers.

It often surprises people to realise how these synthetic vitamins are produced. The individual then has to decide if they are sure that a vitamin produced in this way will be truly identical and have the same actions as a naturally existing vitamin.

Where a vitamin is naturally produced (which is rare) the extraction process itself becomes a potential issue. The effectiveness of isolated vitamins, rather than vitamins found in their natural food sources has been an active debate for many years. The extraction of the vitamin isolates the compound in question from all the other compounds that normally surround it in the natural source. Many of these compounds may actually help increase bioavailability, improve effectiveness and assist detoxification of the product. When removed from its natural food sources the body has to deal with the introduced vitamin compound individually and often in far higher does than would be found in nature. This problem is not unique to Vitamin A and affects many substances extracted from natural food sources.

When examining oral consumption nutritionist universally recommend vitamin rich foods as a better balanced source of vitamins than high dose multivitamins. There is no equivalent advocacy in the cosmetic industry which appears satisfied with mass produced individual synthetic vitamins.

As we will see later there are a variety of different plant based substances that can provide optimum skin nutrition in a wholefood form mirroring the better practices of the oral nutrition industry.

Chapter 8 - How Do You Define Holistic Products?

As discussed above there is no legal definition of natural products. A short dictionary definition refers to natural 'as existing in or formed by nature'[50]. This is not particularly helpful as it is easy to argue what constitutes nature.

For the purpose of this book we are going to define natural products as those existing in nature that have undergone the minimum of human intervention. This definition does not actually create a divide with some products being considered natural and others synthetic, instead it creates a sliding scale with products becoming more natural the less intervention they have undergone.

Unfortunately defining a product as natural is not enough for our purposes. There are a variety of 'natural' products that can be just as harmful if not more so than many synthetic products if consumed.

We therefore have to go a step further and choose products that are truly holistic. By this I mean that as well as being natural they will benefit the person as a whole when used for their correct purpose with the minimum of side effects.

For this purpose I use our Holistic Product pyramid which allows me to quickly decide if the product is holistic and worth exploring further for use with microneedling. Other classification systems may also be useful here and this system just provides one very simple and efficient way to evaluate products.

The Holistic Product Pyramid

The Holistic product pyramid is designed principally to determine 3 things

1. How natural is the product?
2. How safe is the product?
3. How effective is the product?

In many cases you will not be able to meet all criteria but the more the better. I have listed them in approximate order of importance. The most common products that meet these requirements are herbal extracts and specific examples will be provided in the next chapter.

When considering microneedling directly another layer could be added to this pyramid showing a safe history of use as an intramuscular or intradermal injection. This gives another level of assurance that the product will be safe when entering the systemic circulation directly.

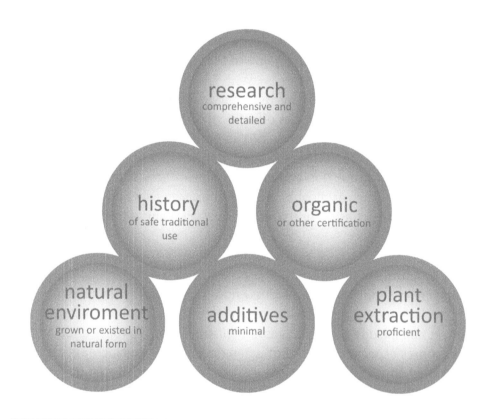

Diagram 2: Holistic Product Pyramid

1. Grown or Existing in a Natural Form in the Natural Environment

By this I simply mean that the substance whether it animal, vegetable or mineral exists in the natural world rather than being a synthetically created chemical in a laboratory. The most common example of these are herbs and other plants used for medicinal or cosmetic purposes. Many animal products would also fit this definition though our clinic has always avoided their use due to ethical considerations and so I have less experience with these substances.

2. Whole Plant Extraction

At present it is impossible to patent a naturally occurring plant. It is however possible to patent a unique chemical isolated from an herb or plant and then reproduced in the laboratory. A patent allows a company exclusive rights to profit from the product for a period of years. For this reason pharmaceutical companies focus their research on isolating one particular chemical with therapeutic effect and then concentrating it. It is then often sold as an extract of the original plant allowing the company to profit from association with the name of the herb.

Many people are unaware of this monetary connection and assume that isolated chemicals must be more effective than the whole plant. Whole herb extractions retain as much as possible the unique chemical balance existing in nature. Often one compound in the herb is balanced by the others improving absorption and reducing side effects. Herbs extracted in a natural solvent such as alcohol or oil are best wherever possible as they are very safe and act as natural preservatives avoiding the addition of unwanted chemicals.

3. Lack of Additives

Although many additives are relatively non-toxic it seems sensible to avoid any unnecessary substances when choosing natural products. Additives can include preservatives, stabilisers, fillers, flavours or colours. This becomes especially important when dealing with the increased transdermal absorption produced by microneedling as we are not currently aware of the effects of most additives when absorbed this way.

4. Organic or Other Certification

Wherever possible we use products that have achieved organic certification. This ensures the products are produced in a more sensitive way and reduces the risks associated with contamination. Due to the cost of certification for the producers (who are often in the third world) this is not possible for all herbs but is important when available.

5. A History of Safe Traditional Use

By this I mean that the herbs or other medicines have been used for hundreds or even thousands of years by traditional societies. This allows people to observe the effects across generations and so observe any longer term consequences. At present, companies attempt to get products to market as quickly as possible. This usually means they undergo several years of safety testing at best. In some cases this has not been long enough with unfortunate consequences.

When choosing traditional products to use with microneedling it is important to focus on products that were used orally, topically and preferably in conjunction with some form of needling such as acupuncture. In our clinic I have focused on products that were used traditionally but which have often also been adapted to hypodermic injections. This provides another level of evidence of their safety and effectiveness when entering the systemic circulation directly.

6. Modern Scientific Research
The addition of modern scientific research to an herbal medicine adds confidence to our belief in its effectiveness and safety. Although relatively few have been thoroughly researched due to the lack of economic incentive it is important to use these herbs wherever possible. This provides additional and important reassurance about the safety and effectiveness of the herbs.

Chapter 9 - Recommended Products

In this section I will discuss in detail several excellent products for use during the treatments. These products are simple to use and can be applied in any clinic or home environment. Later in the book when discussing treatments I will provide several more complicated formulations that can also be used for specific treatments.
The first product discussed is single herb alcohol extract. This is best applied before the microneedling treatment and the microneedling can then dramatically increase its absorption.

When using alcohol tinctures use a supplier you can trust so you can be sure their herbs are either organic or at least comply with Good Agriculture Practice (GAP) and Good Manufacturing Process (GMP). It is also important to ensure that the tincture is of adequate strength. At least a 1:4 blend is recommended and a 1:3 blend is even better.

The use of alcohol on the skin is often debated. It has the disadvantage of dehydrating the skin prior to treatment. In contrast to this it is an excellent carrier for a variety of strong anti aging herbs and being a natural preservative it avoids the addition of other preservatives to the skin as part of many creams and serums. Alcohol is also an excellent cleanser and disinfectant for the skin reducing the risk of infections. If you are a clinician depending on where you are located you may be required to apply alcohol to the skin prior to needling and the strong tinctures make an excellent alternative to isopropyl alcohol.

I do not recommend producing the tinctures in your clinic even if you are trained in this field. The laws surrounding these practices vary from country to country and are particularly strict on clinicians in some countries. It can also affect insurance if for any reason an infection did occur. Good quality tinctures, produced in quality controlled conditions are relatively cheap to purchase and you only require around 2mL per treatment. I now only use tinctures produced in single use ampoules so mirroring some of the better quality and hygiene practices of the cosmetic industry.

The aftercare serum I recommend is actually an oil. The reason for this and its unique properties will be explained in detail below.

Ginseng (*Panax ginseng*) – During the Treatment

Ginseng is a highly effective herb for cosmetic treatments. In Asia it is referred to as the king of herbs. This popularity has led to a huge body of research which can help highlight how Ginseng works for our purposes.

Traditionally it has been used safely both topically and orally for thousands of years. Topically it was used both for anti aging treatments and to assist hair loss. In addition it has also become a common practice to use injections of Ginseng into acupuncture points in hospitals in China. This level of use can provide us with a great deal of assurance of its safety and effectiveness when applied in conjunction with microneedling.

Clinically I use an alcoholic extract of straight red Korean Ginseng prior to microneedling treatments.

The Research on Ginseng
- Produces collagen type 1 when applied topically[51,52].
- Topical extracts of Ginseng increase the transduction of Tat-Cu,Zn-superoxide dismutase (Tat-SOD)[53]. This is a major anti-oxidant enzyme that is showing strong anti aging potential.
- Topically it demonstrates a strong anti-bacterial effect reducing the chances of infection following microneedling treatments[54].
- It can inhibit testosterone 5α-Reductase[13]. High levels of this hormone are increasingly being seen as one of the major causes of hair loss.

It also contains Vitamins A, B-6 and the mineral zinc all of which are considered essential for wound repair but in a natural formulation as an alternative to the synthetic vitamins listed above.

Green tea oil (*Camellia oil*) - Aftercare

Green tea oil is one of the most fascinating anti aging oils currently available. It is made from the seeds of the Camellia genus which are used to produce the world's tea including green tea, oolong tea and even English Breakfast tea. It is quite rare in the Western World often having to be bought on allocation once a year.

Traditionally in Asia it was used both orally for cooking and topically for cosmetic purposes. It was also traditionally applied extensively as a medicine for all forms of skin burns[55]. It has a very long history of use and is a very stable and safe product. Cosmetically it was always considered different to other oils as it did not block the pores. This is a traditional way of saying it does not cause acne. Modern research is now supporting this claim. Oils are very effective moisturisers and would be used more in the cosmetic industry if many did not cause acne in younger skin. This is the major drawback with oils such as Argan and Jojoba oil.

The Research on Green Tea Oil
- The oil is particularly rich in anti-oxidants with at least 9 major anti-oxidant compounds so far having been identified[56].
- The oil contains a high percentage of polyphenols which are some of the most potent and effective anti-oxidant compounds available[56].
- The oil demonstrates strong antimicrobial properties [57].
- Green tea oil has shown strong antiproliferative properties against at least 3 major forms of cancer[56].

Additionally there has been extensive research on the topical application of green tea. Much of the effectiveness of these topical applications in attributed to the polyphenols and linolenic acid which is found in the leaves, stem, bark and seeds of the plant which are used to make green tea oil[56].

- Applied topically green tea is extremely high in anti-oxidants, possessing anti carcinogenic and anti-inflammatory properties, inhibits UV radiation-induced skin carcinogenesis and prevents immunosuppression and oxidative stress[58].
- A recent trial comparing the anti aging properties of topical green tea with 21 herbs popular in European culture for anti aging found the tea extract be nearly twice as effective as its nearest rival[59].
- Topical Green tea ability to prevent UV damage is widely documented. A recent review of 88 scientific studies concluded that it can ameliorate the effects of both UVA and UVB radiation[60]. Some of the most interesting studies showed that topical application prior to exposure inhibits the erythema (redness) response produced by exposure to UV radiation. In addition when studying the histological results it was shown that the topical tea extract reduced the number of sunburnt cells, protected epidermal Langerhans cells from UV damage and reduced the DNA damage that formed after UV radiation[61].

- Topical application of green tea extracts was found to be an effective treatment for radiation induced skin toxicity following the treatment of solid tumours [62]
- Topical Green tea positively influences sebum production in healthy adults[63]. This study concluded that one of the major contributors to the green teas effectiveness was linolenic acid which comprises on average 22.41% of the green tea oil[56].
- Topical use for 6 weeks demonstrated a 58% decrease acne lesions in 20 teenage acne sufferers[64].

Green Tea Oil and Microneedling
Green tea oil is particularly effective following a microneedling treatment for 2 main reasons

1. It has strong anti aging properties which enhance the results of the treatment.
2. It has the ability to reduce the redness, dryness and photosensitivity produced by microneedling.

The anti aging properties are amply explained in the research section below but it is worth understanding how it reduces the side effects of microneedling separately.

The most common side effects of microneedling are;

1. Inflammation (redness)
2. Moisture loss (dryness)
3. Photosensitivity (sensitivity to sunlight).

How green tea oil works to reduce these effects

1. It is a natural anti-inflammatory reducing the redness.
2. Being oil it rapidly moisturises the skin in a way that water based moisturisers cannot.
3. The UV protective property reduces the skins sensitivity to sunlight following treatments.

This provides a stark contrast with many commercially promoted after care products which actually exaggerate the side effects of microneedling.

Clinically I use 100% organic green tea oil containing several herbs that have been macerated into the oil to further improve its effectiveness. Make sure any products you buy are at least 90% green tea oil and are not adding a minute amount of the product simply to be able to add the name to the label. A good indicator of this is the presence of any preservatives or fillers. These are totally unnecessary with green tea oil which is a natural preservative.

Following a treatment I apply the green tea oil quite liberally to the skin. I then supply clients with a small bottle to take home and apply to the face twice a day for the next 2 weeks to reduce the potential side effects listed above and improve the results. Clients need to use as little as 6-8 drops twice a day mixed with a little water to help it spread across the whole face or area being treated.

Providing a natural moisturizer like the green tea oil reduces the reliance on other products which may contain a variety of unfamiliar chemicals which would be absorbed in larger amounts following the microneedling therapy.

Which Products were used as part of the Research Demonstrating the Effectiveness of Microneedling?
An issue with which I are constantly confronted when advocating the use of natural products with microneedling is which products were used during the research demonstrating the effectiveness of microneedling.

Many studies have in fact been done using products like Vitamin A and are sponsored by the companies who produce these products. But several of the best studies have been done using 'dry microneedling' which means no other products were used[29,33]. This includes a 2006 study in which biopsies showed an average collagen increase of 206% and one case of a 1,000% increase[29].

This is not to say that some additional products cannot improve the results of microneedling. I know from my results that I can achieve better results with fewer side effects by using the natural products listed above. It simply states that no products are a necessity for microneedling to work as some advertising would lead you to believe.

Oral Supplementation during Treatment

It is widely recognised that higher nutritional levels can be required during extensive wound healing. The benefit of oral supplementation with the tiny 'wounds' caused by microneedling is debatable. In many clinics that practice more traumatic microneedling techniques a variety of synthetic vitamins, minerals and supplements are prescribed. These can include vitamins A, E and C, the minerals iron, zinc and copper as well as amino acids and omega 3.

The research into the effects of taking synthetic vitamins orally is mixed with some showing good results and some showing negative results bordering on the alarming. Two of the largest and most well-funded recent trials have actually shown large increases in prostate and breast cancer associated with their use[65,66]. The largest of these studies was conducted over 35,329 women.

In clinic I have not found oral supplementation necessary to achieve results with microneedling. However as there may be a potential benefit I usually recommend a natural alternative to these high dose synthetic vitamins. I simply use wholefoods to serve the same purpose as the synthetic vitamins. These wholefoods contain a wide variety of vitamins and minerals essential to the body but in a more balanced, easily assimilated form.

Repeatedly over the last 20 years we have seen vitamin supplement combinations be replaced and updated as it is realised more and more that vitamins and minerals work in synergy. By this I mean that most vitamins and minerals are only absorbed properly when combined with other vitamins and minerals in the correct proportions. The exact combinations required are of course immensely complicated and we are continually updating our knowledge. This research is increasingly showing that products such as wholefoods have already combined these vitamins and minerals in the perfect combination to allow maximum absorption and assimilation of nutrients.

Examples of these wholefood supplements often referred to as super-foods include Spirulina, Chlorella, Wild Blue Green algae, wheat and barley grass. Below we examine spirulina which is perhaps the best all round wholefood to be taken during a course of microneedling treatments.

Spirulina

Spirulina is a microalgae that is used widely as a nutritional supplement. It has a very high protein percentage 85% which is digested compared to only 20% for beef showing how easily the body assimilates it[67]. This protein is made up of all the essential amino acids.

In addition to being high in amino acids Spirulina is very high in a wide range of essential nutrients for wound repair. Of particular interest is the high dose of beta carotene at about 250,000 I.U. per 100 grams[68]. This beta carotene is particularly well converted to vitamin A due to the high levels of chlorophyll which work synergistically with the beta carotene. The chlorophyll activates enzymes that produce vitamin E and K both of which help convert beta carotene into vitamin A. This is a natural form of vitamin A in a small safe dose.

In addition to beta carotene Spirulina contains natural, easily absorbed forms of omega 3, gamma-linolenic acid (GLA), alpha-linolenic acid (ALA), linoleic acid (LA), vitamins B1 (thiamine), B2 (riboflavin), B3 (nicotinamide), B6 (pyridoxine), B9 (folic acid), vitamin C, vitamin D and vitamin E. It is also a source of potassium, calcium, chromium, copper, iron, magnesium, manganese, phosphorus, selenium, sodium and zinc[68].

As you can see Spirulina contains the essentials vitamins and minerals for wound repair but in an easily absorbed wholefood form.

The concentrations of these minerals vary from brand to brand depending on where they are produced so it is best to follow the manufacturers recommended dosage.

A Quick Warning

The chapter above about the use of natural substances is not an invitation to simply apply any apparently natural product to the skin during a microneedling treatment and see what happens. As discussed earlier natural substances can be as greater a health concern as synthetic products if used incorrectly. The substances listed above have a long history of safe and effective internal (oral) use, topical use with acupuncture and where possible recent safe use as intramuscular injections.

Of particular concern here are some essential oils. The method of extraction of essential oils leads to a very high concentration of a limited group of compounds from the plant used. This can be very useful for some purposes but can lead to higher rates of skin reaction when used with microneedling. Many essential oils also have a strong influence on the hormonal system and this effect is only likely to be magnified by the increase in transdermal absorption caused by microneedling. As with any other product they should be assessed on a case by case basis. They should not immediately be assumed to be safe because they are natural. Unless you are really sure about a substance it is best to seek advice before applying it in conjunction with microneedling.

Principle 2 – Use the Least Invasive Microneedling Techniques to Achieve the Desired Results

Overview

Using the least invasive microneedling techniques can be conveniently broken down into three major subjects.

1. Use the shortest possible needles to achieve the desired results.
2. Use good needling or rolling techniques to reduce pain and unnecessary trauma.
3. Use the minimum amount of anaesthetic by minimising pain through correct needle size and technique.

Microneedling achieves results by creating micro trauma within the skin. Although this trauma is minor it is still an injury to the body. In this context it only makes sense to cause the least possible trauma to achieve the maximum results. Some level of trauma is critical to the results but injuring other usually deeper tissues unnecessarily simply does not make sense. It only increases recovery time, discomfort, the number of product that must be used (anaesthetics) and the overall drain on the body's resources. Against this background we need to choose the shortest possible needle length that will achieve results.

Good technique can make the treatments much less painful and either reduce or eliminate the need for anaesthetic all together. Techniques are best taught in person but we can lay out a few simple principles that allow the microneedling treatments to work more closely with the traditional understanding of the body so reducing pain and potential side effects. All techniques are explained in part 3 'Performing Holistic Microneedling Treatments'.

The third concerns the indiscriminate use of anaesthetics. By combining shorter needles with correct technique the need for anaesthetics can usually be eliminated completely. Excessive use of anaesthetics encourages poor quality and lazy techniques. Anaesthetics are necessary in some situations but if they are not necessary then it is better practice not to use them. Our principle here is as discussed to cause the minimum harm for the maximum results. Although the risk with topical anaesthetic is small if their use is unnecessary then it is still an unnecessary risk.

Currently in the west it is rare to find any of these points listed above being practiced. Instead a one size fits all attitude has often been adopted. This is commonly referred to as 'medical skin needling or medical microneedling'. Using these techniques 1.5mm needles or above are used for all purposes regardless of their necessity. This practice combined with slow heavy handed needling technique produces a lot of blood, pain and extensive trauma.

'Medical skin needling' transforms microneedling into a practice that can only be performed in a medically supervised environment due to the obvious risks which accompany this type of treatment. It is reported to be extremely painful and local anaesthetics administered through hypodermic needles are often required in addition to topical anaesthetics to allow patient compliance.

As we will see through the research this is often very unnecessary.

Chapter 10 - Which Needle Length?

The skin varies in thickness from 0.5mm to 4.0mm on the soles of the feet. The average thickness of the skin is 1.5mm. Within the skin are the more superficial epidermis which is 0.10-0.15mm thick and the deeper dermis. The most superficial layer of the epidermis is the stratum corneum which is 0.01 – 0.02 mm thick. Please see diagram 1 if you need to review the structure of the skin.

The appropriate length of microneedle to use depends upon the purpose. Needles as short as 0.15mm are long enough to increase transdermal absorption but are of no use for collagen induction. A 0.5mm long microneedle is the most effective for increasing transdermal absorption and also the shortest needle that will induct collagen. It is undoubtedly the most useful all round microneedle length. Needles longer than this can be used for specific purposes but their use must be weighed against the level of trauma they cause.

There is a growing body of evidence supporting the use of shorter microneedles to achieve similar or better results than longer microneedles. A recent retrospective analysis of 44 patients rated the visual improvement in facial appearance higher with a 0.5mm roller than with a 2.0mm roller[10]. Another well-known study showed that even when using a 1.5mm roller the collagen induction only takes place to a depth of 0.5-0.6mm[29]. It is also important to note that the studies that demonstrate skin thickening show that it occurs in the strateum spinosa again in the superficial epidermis easily reached with a 0.5mm roller[30]. These studies provide supporting evidence for what I have found in clinic. When selecting microneedle length less is often more.

What follows is an explanation of some of the key concepts in choosing an appropriate needle length along with a description of each individual microneedle length, its uses and a quick reference table. Throughout the book I have referred to the needle length in mm where normal practice would be to use micrometers (μm) for the shorter sizes. I will continue this practice here as it avoids confusion for those not familiar with working in μm and avoids having to constantly convert between mm and μm.

Variations in Skin Thickness

A frequently asked question by recipients of microneedle treatments is does the individual thickness of the skin effect how long a microneedle is required? This is a good question as it is well known that the thickness of skin varies from person to person. The main variations in skin thickness occur at the dermis level meaning the epidermis is fairly similar in most people. As the epidermis is so thin anyway at 0.10-0.15mm thick any slight variation is not going to affect your results when using a 0.5mm microneedle or longer. Therefore the same length microneedle is long enough to pass through the epidermis to the dermis to stimulate collagen induction in individuals of different races, sex and sizes.

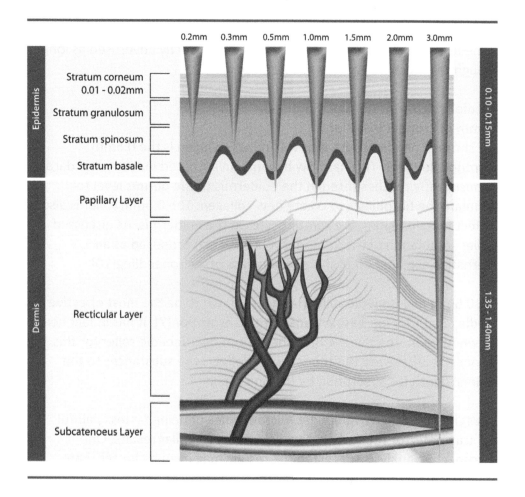

Diagram 3 – Needle Penetration Depth

A Summary of Each Microneedle Length

Needle Lengths for Transdermal Absorption Only
0.15mm – 0.3mm Microneedle Rollers
The stratum corneum is only 0.01 – 0.02 mm thick. Therefore very short microneedles can be used to penetrate this barrier increasing transdermal absorption. The stratum corneum actually contains no nerves. If needles were used that were short enough to only penetrate this barrier but not the deeper tissues the needles would not only be painless but barely felt. However to account for hair, tiny wrinkles and other surface features and to allow a large margin of error rollers containing microneedles of between 0.15mm and 0.3mm in length are usually used when exclusively increasing transdermal absorption. These are sometimes referred to as home use rollers and have previously been incorrectly advertised as long enough to induct collagen by some companies.

Needle Lengths for Collagen Induction
0.5mm Microneedle Roller
The shortest needle length that will induct collagen is the 0.5mm microneedle roller. This has now become an accepted industry standard. It consistently reaches through the epidermis to the dermis level to stimulate the fibroblasts to create new collagen. The 0.5mm roller is also perfect for stimulating the keratinocytes in the epidermis. As discussed earlier stimulation of the keratinocytes has been proposed as an alternative explanation of the effectiveness of microneedling[10].

The 0.5mm microneedle roller has been shown to be the most effective needle length for increasing transdermal absorption[7]. It has in fact been shown to be more effective than the 1.5mm microneedle roller for this purpose. It is believed this is because it delivers the substances to the optimal depth for absorption by the fine capillaries.

It has the advantage over longer microneedles of being far less painful and traumatic for the recipient while achieving similar results. One retrospective analysis suggested the results may even be better than when using a 2.0mm roller[10]. The reduced levels of pain experienced when combined with the correct techniques can allow the roller to be used without anaesthetic which saves time and the addition of another unnecessary chemical product applied to the skin.

The 0.5mm roller is the best all round needle length for anti aging treatments, UV damage, wrinkles, hyperpigmentation, hand rejuvenation, the décolletage, sagging arms and sagging facial skin.

0.75mm Microneedle Roller
Although the 0.5mm roller is generally my first choice where stronger stimulation is required I select the 0.75mm roller. This roller is a preferred choice in cases of mild facial acne scarring. Studies have shown that even when using the 1.5mm roller collagen induction only takes place up to 0.6mm in depth. By using the 0.75mm roller it is easy to cover this entire depth with a large margin of error.

1.0mm Microneedle Roller
This is a less used needle length. It can be of assistance when working with hair loss as the extra length allows it to pass through the cushioning provided by any hair in the area. It is also sometimes useful for assisting facial scars.

1.5mm Microneedle Roller
The 1.5mm roller is most useful for treating more severe scarring, stretch marks and cellulite. The 0.5mm roller is generally slower to break up the knotted collagen bundles of larger scars and stretch marks. This length is also useful to benefit cellulite. The exact mechanism by which it does this remains unknown. However our clinical experience has found that shorter needles like the 0.5mm although effective are not as fast acting as the 1.5mm needles in cases of cellulite.

There are several companies who deal principally with doctors and highly trained medical professionals which only recommend the 1.5mm roller and longer for all purposes. As discussed previously many of the earlier microneedle rollers used by the medical profession were 3.0mm long and were so painful they had to be applied in a hospital setting. There has since been a progression to shorter needles. If the same or even better results can be achieved with a shorter less invasive microneedle then using a 1.5mm needle may just be causing unnecessary structural damage.

Where there is severe scarring on the face it can be a good idea to use the 1.5mm roller. This is generally performed with a topical anaesthetic and is highly recommended to be done by a clinician rather than at home as it will cause pain and bleeding. If using the 1.5mm microneedles aftercare also becomes more important as the deeper penetration also has increased risk of infection though this is extremely rare even when compared to the use of hypodermic needles[69].

2.0mm Microneedle Roller
These rollers are only for highly trained and experienced practitioners and can only be used with effective anaesthetic. Topical anaesthetic may not be enough in these cases. I do not recommend the use of this length needle as we have not found any additional benefits when used in clinic. The best use of this needle size is by plastic surgeons who often use the products for severe burn scars and other conditions which are more medical than cosmetic.

3.0mm Microneedle Roller
Keep in mind that the skin is only an average of 1.5mm thick so if used with strong pressure the 3.0mm needles will definitely pass through the dermis into the subcutaneous layer separating the dermis from the structures below. There are no fibroblasts in this area and unnecessary damage is usually being done.

Dermastamp
This is, as the name suggests, a small stamp with microneedles attached. It lacks the rolling action which smoothly inserts the needles and is therefore far less popular.

It is however often a better option when treating hair loss for patients who still have reasonable length hair in the treatment area. The issue with the roller is that hair sometimes gets caught in the axel and is pulled out. This is counter-productive and very distressing to see further hair being removed. In these cases of hair loss I use a 1.0mm needle length dermastamp as the extra length is required to overcome the cushioning effect of the hair.

The dermastamp can also be useful for small isolated scars where rolling will simply cover a larger and unnecessary area of skin. Its action is more abrupt and less smooth than the roller but it can be very effective. As most scars treated in this way tend to be very small a 1.0mm dermastamp is usually quite long enough.

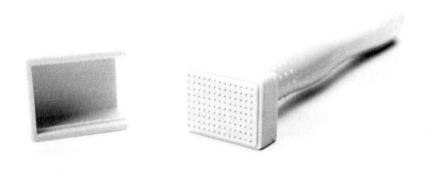

Image 7: 1.0mm Dermastamp

Needle Length Reference Table

Needle Length	Indications
0.15-0.3mm	Increases transdermal absorption
0.5mm	Collagen induction, anti aging, wrinkles, UV damage, hyperpigmentation, non pustular/non nodular rosacea, thin skin, enlarged pores, skin laxity, sagging skin, sagging upper arms, hand rejuvenation, age spots, inactive acne
0.75mm	Shallow facial scars, anti aging, hair loss
1.0mm	Hair loss,
1.5mm	Severe scarring, stretch marks, cellulite
2.0mm	Highly trained medical use only
3.0mm	Best avoided or very specific medical use
1.0mm dermastamp	Hair loss, small isolated scars

Principle 3 – Apply the Principles of Traditional Medicine to Improve Microneedling Treatments

Chapter 11 - Why Apply a Traditional Medicine System?

Throughout this book it has been demonstrated how successfully microneedling can be transformed into a completely holistic treatment. By adapting it into a traditional medicine system you provide a framework within which it can be adapted to a wide variety of different conditions and situations. It then benefits from thousands of years of first-hand experience. In essence what you are doing is borrowing a readymade holistic philosophy complete with treatment principles and protocols into which microneedling can easily be incorporated.

My own early training was in Traditional Chinese Medicine (TCM) so this was the system I naturally adapted. There are however a number of other reasons to apply the principles of TCM to Holistic Microneedling.

1. TCM was the original form of cosmetic skin needling. This means that many of the practices have already been tested for hundreds of years in slightly different forms.
2. TCM is a completely holistic therapy which recognises the person as a whole and recognises the constant interactions going on between all parts of the body. It provides an excellent way of overcoming the segmental view of the body often adopted by the cosmetic industry.
3. In addition to therapeutic medicine TCM has a long and distinguished history of holistic cosmetic treatments from which to borrow ideas. This can enhance treatments and allow you to add other natural treatments to the holistic microneedling treatment.

The Traditional Chinese Understanding of Beauty
The Chinese understanding of the body was very different to our current anatomical definition. There was a belief that in addition to anatomy the body was in fact supported by energy or qi as the Chinese call it. To oversimplify slightly the healthier a person was the more qi they currently possessed. Some activities enhanced qi and some detracted from it.

The ancient Chinese understanding of beauty was that it was simply a reflection of healthy qi. Therefore beauty and health were inseparable. No cosmetic practices were performed that damaged the health and therefore qi of the individual. This included excessively wounding the body as bleeding was draining to qi and blood and scar tissue was considered very detrimental to health. These beliefs would largely eliminate our cosmetic surgery industry and several of our non-surgical cosmetic practices if applied today.

The aim of TCM was always to prevent illness and so encourage health which was synonymous with beauty. The motivation of Chinese doctors was very strong as patients paid the doctor a retainer when they were healthy and the payment ceased if they were unwell, only recommencing when the doctor could restore their health. This clearly demonstrates the Chinese concept that prevention and maintenance were better than dramatic intervention later.

This was applied equally to their cosmetic system where in addition to skin needling subtle tools like the jade roller were employed daily to prevent the signs of aging. Wealthy families slept on silk not simply because they could afford it but because they realised that it formed a barrier with the skin preventing the leaching of moisture over-night and preventing asymmetrical wrinkle formation on the side of the face more often slept on. These wrinkles are common with cotton pillow cases.

Men also realised that silk did not produce friction and so did not tear out already thinning hair overnight while they slept. Traditional Chinese herbal formulas were employed topically to the skin to prevent the signs of aging. Physicians to important women of ancient China spent no less time developing their herbal beauty creams than modern researchers. Their orientation was simply different in that they believed it had to enhance the health at all levels to achieve results.

A fascinating example of the way health and beauty interacts in the TCM understanding is the way scars were treated. Scar treatments are very popular in the western world for their aesthetic improvement. The Ancient Chinese went beyond this. They were concerned about the visual appearance of a scar and the distress this could cause but they were also equally concerned with the location of the scar and which acupuncture meridians the scar may be interrupting. TCM understands that the body's qi flows in these meridians. A scar across one of these meridians can interrupt the healthy flow of qi and ultimately lead to illness which further damages beauty.

Treatments involving topical herbs as well as skin needling were developed to directly treat these scars which were seen as a serious problem (Please see the earlier picture of the circling the dragon technique). Acupuncturists today still pay very close attention to the location of scars and which meridian and therefore internal organs they may be affecting. Scars from gynaecological surgery are treated very seriously as this area is very rich in acupuncture meridians and illnesses in this area can easily develop.

Another striking example was the development of Chinese Medical Face Reading. This system simply identified the location of each wrinkle or blemish on the face and related it back to the internal organ that was understood to control that area. For example, deep lines from the corner of the nose down to the corners of the mouth were understood to indicate issues with the large intestine or Gall bladder. Although no longer popular it is hard to imagine a system that more closely connected the idea of health and beauty.

Current cosmetic practices do not reflect this philosophy that all treatments should enhance health. Currently as long as a treatment does not produce immediate symptoms it is considered safe. No consideration is given to the subtle changes we may be producing or the future consequences of the treatments. Applying the ancient TCM philosophy to modern microneedling allows us to develop practices which enhance health and minimise unnecessary damage while still achieving results.

Applying the Acupuncture Meridians to Microneedling
During my early training all cosmetic treatments I learned were applied with respect to the natural flow of qi in the acupuncture meridians. The idea is to work with the body to achieve the aesthetic results rather than against it by sheer brute force.

The acupuncture meridians consist of pathways through which it is traditionally considered the body's energy flow. These pathways are too small to be detected by a microscope but can be observed either through their electrical resistance or in one unique experiment by injecting radioactive technetium into acupuncture points in the body and using nuclear scanning equipment to watch its flow along the acupuncture meridian[70,71]. For our purposes it is important to note that the pathways all flow in one direction only.

The knowledge of their existence dates back at least 2,000 years and is probably much older. In TCM the flow in these channels is regulated and often corrected by the use of acupuncture needles. Additionally, massage and other manipulation techniques are often applied in the direction of the channel flow to enhance health and beauty.

Wherever possible, microneedling should be applied in the direction of the acupuncture channels in that area. This involves no inconvenience as treatments are completed just as quickly and rolling in only one direction has other advantages that will be discussed shortly. It is just as easy to provide full surface coverage of the skin being treated and the microneedling is then starting to work with the body's natural flow rather than against it.

In addition to the acupuncture meridians ancient cosmetic treatments also followed certain principles that were shown to enhance results. The most obvious examples of this are on the face where it is very difficult to follow every acupuncture channel directly. The principles then followed are;

1. Always start treatments on the right side of the face and treat the left side afterwards as this is the direction the qi flows in this area.
2. Start in the centre of the face and roll outwards, never inwards as this stretches and tightens the skin.
3. Wherever possible roll upwards as this lifts the qi in the area and prevents sagging.

Interestingly applying these techniques takes no more time or effort than modern techniques. It also works perfectly with the contours of the face and in my experience produces far superior results.

Individualised Treatments
A natural progression of treating every person as a whole is acknowledging that every individual is different. TCM has always customised its cosmetic and therapeutic treatments to the individual's

constitution. One size fits all treatments were simply not part of the Chinese culture. Each individual was recognised as different and an individual formula of herbs or individual acupuncture points selected to benefit that individual.

The modern cosmetic approach to microneedling could be summarised by the phrase 'skin is skin'. All skin is assumed to respond to exactly the same substances and treated exactly the same way. There is no recognition that there is an individual person attached to the skin who may respond differently based on their constitution which is reflected in their skin type.

By applying the theories of TCM to microneedling treatments can become tailor made as they are designed to benefit exactly the individual being treated. This customisation can take place, in the herbs used on the skin, the treatment times, needle length used, areas treated and the actual treatment techniques used.

A simple example of this is the treatment of older skin. Medical skin needling will treat older skin exactly the same as younger skin. In holistic microneedling it is recognised that older skin is often more sensitive. Different herbal extracts can be applied, shorter treatment times applied and fewer needle insertions used. These are exactly the same principles that are applied to cosmetic acupuncture treatments for older or frailer patients.

Simple Steps to Apply TCM Theory to a Microneedling Treatment
1. Use the least invasive techniques possible. Excessive trauma damages qi and blood.
2. Follow the flow of qi allowing you to work with the body rather than trying to overcome it.
3. Enhance the treatments with natural time tested herbs that can benefit the skin and the individual in the long run.
4. Customise the treatment to the individual wherever possible. Avoid the one size fits all paradigm adopted by the cosmetic industry.

Part 3 - Putting it All Together – Performing Holistic Microneedling Treatments

Chapter 12 - Prior to Treatment

Before you begin the microneedling treatments there are a number of points of which you should be aware. Below is a list of cautions and contraindications that must be observed.

Clinicians performing microneedling treatments for the first time need to ensure that they have adequate insurance in place. They will also need to ask all clients to complete a signed consent form and a client consultation form. This is particularly important as it allows the clinician to identify any contraindications that the client may not otherwise mention. Standard consultation forms are usually acceptable but it is better to use a form specifically designed for microneedling where possible.

Particular note should be made of patients suffering any form of auto immune disease, diabetes or immune suppressed patients as they are at higher risk of infection following treatment.

Cautions and Contraindications

Skin Conditions
- Any open skin wounds including broken skin, scabs, wounds, bleeding skin and blisters should be avoided.
- Cold sores must be avoided if present or they may be spread. If there is a history of cold sores it is often best to begin taking any cold sore medicine before beginning microneedling as any form of skin needling can activate the immune system and cause an outbreak of cold sores. The more aggressive the treatment the greater the likelihood of an outbreak.
- Pustular acne spots should be avoided. Microneedling can actually benefit acne but it is important to treat the area in between outbreaks or treat around open acne spots or you may spread the bacteria. Large acne spots will also be painful to roll across and this should be avoided.
- Rashes, psoriasis, eczema, pustular or nodular rosacea and fungal infections should all be avoided.

- Contagious skin conditions should be avoided.
- Raised moles, warts or moles that have changed shape or colour and unidentified skin growths should be examined by a physician before being treating.
- Bruised skin can be painful to treat and should be avoided.
- Skin cancers must be avoided.
- Keloid scars are also a strict contraindication.

Medications
- Anti coagulation medications present a challenge. Anti-coagulant medications and their interactions are becoming increasingly difficult to monitor. If a client or home user is taking anti-coagulant medication they should consult their prescribing physician before proceeding. Individuals who are taking a low dose of aspirin can usually proceed with the microneedling without adverse effects.
- Any medications that cause photosensitivity should be avoided during courses of microneedling treatments. Some common classes of drugs that may need to be avoided include; Accutane, NSAIDS, some antibiotics, some antidepressants, some antihistamines, some diuretics and some antihypertensives. This list is far from exhaustive and avoids brand names as they vary from country to country. It is best to check the side effects of any medications being taken to ensure they do not cause photosensitivity.
- Areas where topical medication is being applied should be avoided as the increase in transdermal absorption can affect the timing, and quantity of doses absorbed.

Cosmetic Treatments
In addition I suggest microneedling not be performed after a variety of other cosmetic treatments such as microdermabrasion, botulinum toxin, filler injections, IPL, chemical peels or cosmetic surgery until all signs of inflammation caused by the other treatments have passed. For more information on this please see the earlier chapter comparing microneedling to conventional cosmetic treatments.

Other Considerations
- Pregnant women should only receive dry needling (microneedling with no additional products) and I prefer not to treat pregnant

women at all as the body's resources are rightly allocated elsewhere during this time. Besides most pregnant women look particularly young and healthy at this stage due to hormone release and the treatment may be better saved until after the birth.

- Haemophiliacs are a strict contraindication.
- People with a history of allergies such as asthma of hay fever should be warned of an increased risk of urticaria or itchy skin following treatment due to the release of histamines.
- Diabetes is not a strict contraindication if it is controlled but the skin should be closely monitored after treatment due to the higher risk of infection.
- Immune suppressed individuals should be treated on a case by case basis. People suffering from a suppressed immune system should avoid unsupervised microneedling at home.
- Individuals with Fitzpatrick III and above can be treated with microneedling but must be very careful to avoid sun exposure following the treatments and be aware that the inflammation of the skin can appear darker on the skin for several months following treatment. This treatment is best performed under clinical supervision rather than at home.

Treatment Schedule

Treatments should be performed no more than once every 14 days if using a 0.5mm microneedle roller or above. Although I have seen very good results by using 0.5mm rollers more often than this it seems wise to be more cautious and use the rollers consistently over a longer period of time. This allows you to work gently with the body and achieve consistent long term results.

The reason for only treating every 14-30 days is that the levels of collagenase peak around 14 days and then begin to decrease. Collagenase are enzymes that break down existing collagen and are part of the reason microneedling is so effective in assisting scar tissue. I prefer to wait until after it has peaked before initiating the wound healing cycle again.

It is best to do treatments in packages of 6 and then take a break for at least 2 months before beginning treatment again.

Using the rollers more often than this is very tempting, especially for those using them at home. It can produce fast results but can potentially leave the skin in a semi-permanent state of inflammation during the treatment period. This is not beneficial for the underlying health and so I prefer to use is more regularly over a longer period than in quick enthusiastic bursts.

Individuals who are performing more aggressive microneedling techniques as advocated by some companies may have to leave longer gaps between treatments as the inflammation may last longer. This is also the case if using vitamin A creams which I do not recommend as they can also prolong the inflammation and cause additional side effects.

Cleansing the Skin to be Treated
For clinicians the regulations that need to be followed vary from country to country and it is best to follow your local skin penetration guidelines. Below I have listed a simple procedure I use in clinic which can also be replicated easily at home for home users.

1. Cleanse the skin thoroughly using a good quality organic cleanser. Make sure to remove all make up and sunburn cream that may be present.
2. Then apply alcohol to the skin. In clinic I use the high concentration herbal tinctures described in the next sections for this process. If you are not using these tinctures or the legal requirements where you practice require you to use isopropyl alcohol then you must follow this process. This can be in the form of swabs which are easily obtainable from a pharmacy for home users.

Chapter 13 - Performing Microneedling Treatments

Rolling Techniques
1. Hold the roller gently, undue pressure is not required.
2. Only roll the microneedle roller in one direction pulling the drum towards the handle rather than pushing the drum first.
3. Use short strokes to cover the area as quickly as possible
4. Follow the direction of the acupuncture channels or the flow of qi in each area (These are demonstrated shortly).

Explanation of the Techniques
1. Good quality sharp needles will penetrate the skin quickly and easily. Undue pressure will only increase nerve sensitivity and increase the perception of pain. If you find you are using a roller that feels like it is dragging or catching on the skin then the needles are most likely blunt and bent and you need to replace the roller.
2. By dragging rather than pushing the roller you allow the roller to better compensate for the bumps and unevenness of the skin. It is also easier to avoid rolling into protrusions like the nose which can be very painful. Rolling in one direction works with the body' natural qi flow producing a better result. Only rolling in one direction has the additional advantage that the roller is never rolled over exactly the same patch of skin on the same angle again. When the roller is rolled back and forth the needles can reinsert into the same holes again and again. This creates what are called track marks on the skin which are unsightly and take some time to heal. This is easy to avoid by using the correct technique.
3. Using short strokes works better with the contours of the face as it is hard to keep even pressure with longer strokes. When performing longer strokes there is also the tendency to change direction and so drag the needles causing pain.
4. This has been discussed previously and will be explained for each individual area of the body.

Additional Products used with the Treatments
When treating clients in addition to the herbal products listed earlier I use a range of different tinctures and after care serums. These are combinations I have found highly beneficial and extremely safe in on-going clinic use over the years. The method and key ingredients of each

one are listed below so users can gain an understanding of the exact ingredients.

Every herb listed has a long history of safe oral and topical use. Most have also been safely used as hypodermic injections in China for a variety of conditions. I have used all of these combinations in clinic with skin needling for almost a decade now with excellent results and no major side effects. When describing the treatment of each different condition I refer to one of the combinations listed below.

Treatment Tinctures

These are prepared in an organic 1:3 ethanol extract. Alcoholic tinctures have a long history of topical use in China. It is best to ensure that ensure that any tinctures used exceed the British Herbal Pharmacopeia (BHP) by 30%. It is also important that at no time is heat used during the extraction process as this may damage heat sensitive components of the plants such as glycosides and saponins. Good quality tinctures should have High Pressure Liquid Chromatography (HPLC) performed on the finished products to test for purity and marker compounds.

Anti Aging Tincture – *Panax ginseng* (Ginseng), *Ganoderma lucidum* (Ling Zhi or Rei Shi), *Rhodiola rosea* (Rose root)

This is a combination of traditional tonic herbs which have been extensively researched for their anti aging properties. They influence wound healing, collagen and elastin production and contain powerful antioxidants.

Scar and Stretch Marks Tincture – *Panax notoginseng* (San Qi), *Rhodiola rosea* (Rose Root), *Olibannum gummi* (Ru Xiang)

These herbs are a combination of tonics and herbs specifically used to increase blood circulation in traditional understanding. They have been extensively researched and are very useful here as both scars and stretch marks are associated with blood stagnation in TCM philosophy. This is a very simple but effective combination.

Cellulite Tincture – *Panax notoginseng* (San Qi), *Cinnamomum cassia bark* (Rou Gui or Cinnamon)

This is a combination of blood circulating herbs and warming herbs. Traditionally warming herbs were used to assist conditions like cellulite in TCM as cellulite was associated with cold and stagnation in the tissues.

Clear Skin Tincture – *Rheum palmatum root* (Da Huang or Rhubarb), *Camellia sinensis* (White tea), *Olibannum gummi* (Ru Xiang)

These herbs are traditionally used to reduce inflammation and white tea is one of the most powerful anti aging and anti-oxidant herbs so far researched. This combination is very effective against acne and can also be used in cases of rosacea.

Aftercare Serums
These are prepared by professional maceration of the herbs in organic Camellia (green tea) oil. Please read the earlier chapter to learn more about the benefits of green tea oil.

Anti Aging Aftercare Serum – *Camellia oil* (Green tea oil), *Panax ginseng* (Ginseng), *Astragalus membranaceus* (Huang Qi), *Lycium Chinese Fruit* (Gou Ji Berry)

This unique combination of well researched tonic herbs is highly effective at increasing the anti aging effects of the microneedling while the Camellia oil minimises the side effects of dryness and photosensitivity.

Scar Aftercare Serum – *Camellia oil* (Green Tea Oil), *Panax notoginseng* (San Qi), *Commiphora molmol* (Mo Yao or Myrrh), *Carthimus tinctorius* (Hong Hua or Safflower), *Olibannum gummi* (Ru Xiang)

This is a specialised combination of circulating herbs in Camellia oil to reduce the appearance of scars and minimise the dryness and photosensitivity caused by microneedling.

Stretch Mark and Cellulite Aftercare Serum – *Camellia oil* (Green Tea Oil), *Psoralea corylifolia fruit* (Bu Gu Zhi), *Cinnamomum cassia bark* (Rou Gui or Cinnamon), *Panax notoginseng* (San Qi), Ze Lan, *Rheum palmatum root* (Da Huang or Rhubarb)

This is a powerful combination of herbs used to warm the tissues and increase circulation. It is combined with lesser known herbs such as Ze Lan which is specifically used to eliminate water retention in the skin in this formula.

Aftercare Hair Restoration Spray
This is best used as a 1:3 tincture in organic ethanol.
Organic ethanol, *Panax notoginseng* (San Qi), *Polygonum multiflorum* (He Shou Wu), *Zingiber officinate* (Sheng Jiang or Ginger), *Panax ginseng* (Ginseng)

These herbs have been used in China for hundreds of years to assist a variety of different types of hair loss.

On the next couple of pages are listed details of procedures for treating different parts of the body. There is a detailed table at the end of the chapter summarising all these techniques if further information is required.

Microneedling Techniques

Techniques for Treating the Face

1. Cleanse the face thoroughly using a natural cleanser.
2. Apply the Anti Aging tincture using a cotton pad or cleanse with a swab.
3. Select a 0.5mm roller or a longer needle size if treating scarring (see previous section)
4. Start on the right side of the Face. Complete the right side and then do the left.
5. Roll first outwards across the lower jaw from the centre of the chin towards the lower ear.
6. Use short strokes and make sure you overlap each section of the face you do so as not to miss any areas.
7. Continue to place the roller slightly higher up the cheek each time and then roll out towards the ear until you have rolled across the entire chin and cheek in an outwards direction. Avoid the central column of the nose and upper lip at this stage.
8. When rolling outwards below the eyes do not roll into the eye socket to treat fine lines. Instead use the other hand to pull this skin down slightly so that it is resting on the upper cheek bone and then roll across it there.
9. Now roll across the entire section you have just covered in an upwards direction. Be careful not to roll onto the lips when rolling the chin. It is often a good idea to tuck in the lips when doing this section.
10. When rolling upwards on the upper cheek make sure to stop well before the eye.
11. Make sure you roll upwards intently across the crow's feet area, near the temples just outside the eye.
12. Then Roll outwards across the eyebrow. It is important to use the other hand to draw the skin in this area upwards and then roll slightly below the brow so that you are actually working on the skin of the upper eyelid without rolling into the eye socket.
13. Start just above the nose and roll outwards from the centre across the forehead slowly working your way upwards until the entire forehead is covered.
14. Start just above the nose and roll up the forehead. Work your way outwards until you have rolled upwards across the entire right side of the forehead.

15. Roll intently across the area between the eyebrows in an upwards direction varying the direction slightly from straight up to 45 degrees.
16. At this point if special attention is required on the nasolabial lines (corner of the nose to the corner of the mouth) you can roll down these.
17. Repeat the entire procedure on the left side of the face.
18. Return to the nose and roll down the nose including the centre and both sides.
19. Tuck the lips in and roll outwards across the gap between the nose and mouth. Start at the centre and do the right side and then the left.
20. Roll across each area 10-15 times before moving on. Do count each roll as it is easy to lose track.
21. Apply the Anti Aging aftercare serum liberally across the face.
22. Follow the aftercare advice and avoid bright sunlight wherever possible for several days. If bright sunlight is unavoidable then high quality SPF 30+ sunscreen should be applied.
23. Continue to apply the Anti Aging aftercare serum twice a day for 2 weeks after treatment.

Notes for Treating the Face

1. Always roll upwards and outwards on the face lifting and tightening the skin.
2. Do not use the redness of the skin as a guide that an area has been covered correctly. The skin continues to become flushed for 20 minutes after treatment and may not immediately become red. Do not keep rolling until it is red! You may be surprised how colourful the skin is 20 minutes later. Bear in mind that not all skin types will become red and this is not necessary to achieve results.
3. There are 2 exceptions where we roll downwards in the above treatment. This is simply due to the anatomy of the face. In 95% of techniques rolling upwards and outwards is actually the most effective way to work with the face.
4. The central column of the nose and upper lip are treated last as these can be more painful and so are best left until the treatment is almost finished.
5. Treating the nose last for people who suffer sinus issues is also a good idea as microneedling can cause sneezing (Move the roller away rapidly if sneezing is imminent!).

6. When treating above and below the eyes it is important to stretch the skin away from the eyes rather than roll into the eye socket. This allows the area to be treated correctly but avoids any risk.

7. When rolling on the face of clients it is important to ask them to close their eyes as a close up view of the needles is often disconcerting.

8. Clinicians may need to ask clients to roll their heads to the side to allow easier access to the periphery of the face.

9. There is a cosmetic acupuncture treatment which can be applied to the edge of the lips in which needles are deliberately inserted repeatedly to this area. This creates swelling for a period of 3-5 days and produces a look similar to the collagen injections into the lips which were popular in the 1990's. Microneedling can achieve similar results, but as this look is no longer popular it is best avoided.

10. If assisting very mild acne or non pustular/ non nodular rosacea then the same techniques can be used on the face but the clear skin tincture should be used instead of the Anti Aging tincture.

11. If assisting facial scarring then the same techniques can be applied but a 0.75mm or 1.5mm needle length should be selected depending on the severity of the scars.

12. Be careful when rolling around the hair line not to allow hair to become entangled in the roller and pulled out.

13. If applying sunscreen ensure it is high quality and fresh. Old and dirty sunscreens can increase the chances of developing a rash or skin infection following microneedling.

Directions for the Face

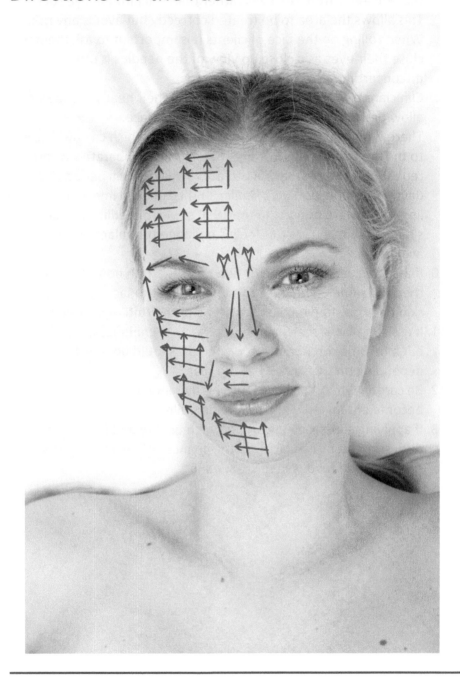

Techniques for Treating the Neck

1. Cleanse the neck thoroughly using a natural or organic cleanser.
2. Apply the Anti Aging tincture using a cotton pad or cleanse with a swab. It is particularly important to do this thoroughly on the neck
3. Select a 0.5mm roller.
4. Start from the base of the neck in the centre
5. Roll up the whole neck to the jaw line.
6. Slowly move across to the right hand side repeating on each area 10-15 times.
7. Start from the centre at the base of the neck. Roll outwards. Begin each roll slightly higher up the neck until you have covered the whole area with short strokes.
8. Repeat on the left hand side
9. Apply the Anti Aging aftercare serum liberally.
10. Follow the aftercare advice and avoid bright sunlight wherever possible for several days. If bright sunlight is unavoidable then high quality SPF 30+ sunscreen should be applied.
11. Continue to apply the Anti Aging aftercare serum twice a day for 2 weeks after treatment.

Notes for Treating the Neck

1. The neck is a highly sensitive area. Unlike the face it is highly prone to small infections and rashes. For this reason I do not recommend treating the neck unless really necessary. It should also be treated with severe caution by those suffering from diabetes and compromised immune systems.
2. It is important to only use a 0.5mm roller in this area due to the sensitive structures lying below the skin.
3. It should be noted that the adams apple area can be sensitive in men and should be avoided in those with tight skin in the area.
4. If performing this treatment it can often be combined with a facial treatment as they use the same microneedle length, treatment tincture and aftercare serum ingredients.
5. If applying sunscreen ensure it is high quality and fresh. Old and dirty sunscreens can increase the chances of developing a rash or skin infection following microneedling. This is particularly important on the neck which is at higher risk of developing rashes.

Techniques for Treating the Décolletage
1. Cleanse the décolletage thoroughly using a natural or organic cleanser.
2. Apply the Anti Aging tincture using a cotton pad or cleanse with a swab.
3. Select a 0.5mm roller
4. Start from the lower midline and roll upwards.
5. Move slowly across to the right until the entire right hand side has been covered in this way.
6. Then start at the lower section of the midline and roll outwards covering the entire area.
7. Gradually move upwards covering the entire right hand side.
8. Repeat the process on the left hand side.
9. Repeat each step 10-15 times
10. Apply the Anti Aging aftercare serum liberally to the area.
11. Follow the aftercare advice and avoid bright sunlight wherever possible for several days. If bright sunlight is unavoidable then high quality SPF 30+ sunscreen should be applied.
12. Continue to apply the Anti Aging aftercare serum twice a day for 2 weeks after treatment.

Notes for Treating the Décolletage
1. If performing this treatment in clinic male clinicians have to be respectful of the privacy of clients and explain fully what they are doing.
2. If performing this treatment it can often be combined with a facial or neck treatments as they use the same microneedle length and similar treatment tincture and aftercare serum ingredients

Directions for the Neck and Décolletage

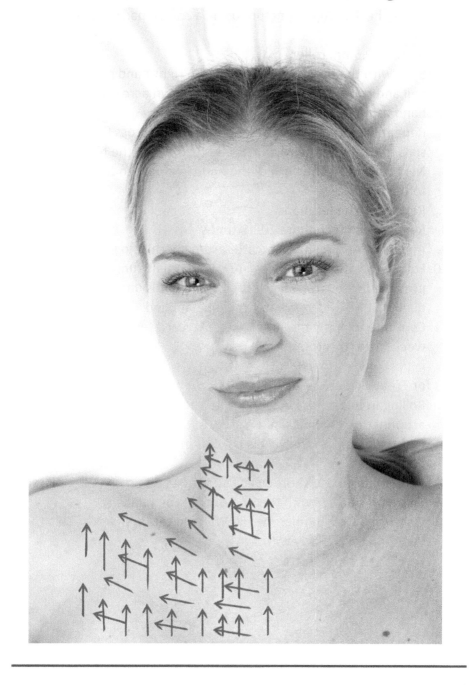

Techniques for Treating the Hands

1. Cleanse the hands thoroughly using a natural or organic cleanser.
2. Apply the Anti Aging tincture using a cotton pad or cleanse with a swab.
3. Select a 0.5mm roller
4. Start with the tip of the thumb on the right hand proximal to the nail and roll up the entire thumb and down across the back of the hand using short strokes.
5. Repeat this practice on each of the fingers across the hand. Make sure to continue the roll up across the back of the hands.
6. Next roll across the back of the hand in a perpendicular direction to the fingers.
7. Repeat on the left hand
8. Repeat each technique 10-15 times.
9. Apply the Anti Aging aftercare serum liberally to the area.
10. Follow the aftercare advice and avoid bright sunlight wherever possible for several days. If bright sunlight is unavoidable then high quality SPF 30+ sunscreen should be applied.
11. Continue to apply the Anti Aging aftercare serum twice a day for 2 weeks after treatment.

Notes for Treating the Hands

1. Rolling in this direction works with the direction of the acupuncture channels in the area.
2. It also works with the valves in veins in the body to prevent blood pooling.
3. Remember to use short rolling strokes as depicted in the diagram. This works better with the anatomy of the hand.
4. Only use a 0.5mm microneedle roller in this area as the skin can be very thin particularly with age.

Directions for the Hands

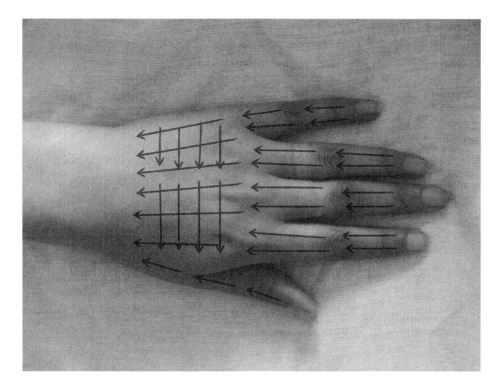

Techniques for Treating the Abdomen
1. Cleanse the abdomen thoroughly using a natural or organic cleanser.
2. Apply the stretch Mark or Scar tincture as appropriate or simply cleanse with a swab.
3. Select a 0.75mm or a 1.5mm microneedle roller
4. Start in the centre on the lower part of the abdomen and roll upwards across the area being treated. Move gradually across to the right until the entire right hand side of the abdomen has been treated.
5. Start in the centre on the lower part of the abdomen and roll outwards from the centre across the right hand side of the area being treated gradually moving upwards over the area being treated.
6. Repeat on the left side.
7. Roll across each area 10-15 times before moving on.

8. Apply the Stretch Mark or Scar aftercare serum liberally to the area.
9. Follow the aftercare advice and avoid bright sunlight wherever possible for several days. If bright sunlight is unavoidable then high quality SPF 30+ sunscreen should be applied.
10. Continue to apply the appropriate aftercare serum twice a day for 2 weeks after treatment.

Notes for Treating the Abdomen
1. For severe stretch marks I recommend a 1.5mm roller as due to the underlying weakness causing the marks they respond more quickly to the longer needles.
2. For smaller scars a 0.75mm microneedle roller is often the better choice.
3. 0.5mm rollers can still achieve results in these cases but work more slowly due to the level of scar tissue that must be broken down.
4. Avoiding the sun is usually easier on the abdomen than the face and hands and direct sunlight should still be avoided for at least 24 hours and ideally several days.
5. If performing this treatment in clinic male clinicians have to be respectful of the privacy of clients and explain fully what they are doing.

Directions for the Abdomen

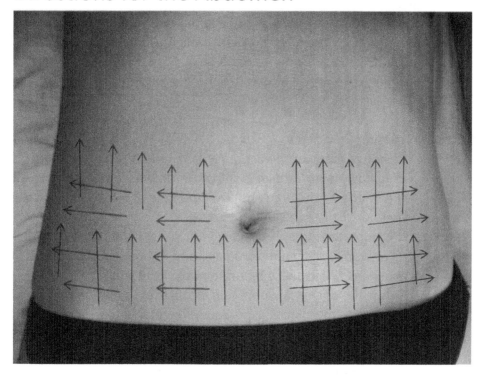

Techniques for Treating the Thighs

1. Cleanse the thigh area thoroughly using a natural or organic cleanser.
2. Apply the Stretch Mark or Cellulite tincture as appropriate or simply cleanse with a swab.
3. Select a 1.5mm microneedle roller
4. Apply a vigorous massage to the thigh area to be treated working upwards towards the body. This area often suffers from poor circulation and the massage will increase the blood flow in the area prior to treatment.
5. Start on the front of the right thigh and roll upwards across the area being treated. Move gradually across to the back of the thigh repeating the technique.
6. Roll outwards from the front of the thigh directly to the back of the thigh across the area being treated gradually moving upwards.
7. Repeat on the left thigh.
8. Roll across each area 10-15 times before moving on.

9. Apply the Stretch Mark or Cellulite aftercare serum liberally to the area.
10. Follow the aftercare advice and avoid bright sunlight wherever possible for several days. If bright sunlight is unavoidable then high quality SPF 30+ sunscreen should be applied.
11. Continue to apply the aftercare serum twice a day for 2 weeks after treatment.

Notes for Treating the Thighs
1. Although many of the acupuncture meridians that cross this area flow downwards it is still preferable to roll upwards to lift the energy in the area and avoid pooling of blood and qi in the feet.
2. It is important to only massage upwards towards the trunk so as to work with venous drainage and not damage the valves in the veins which cause blood to pool in the limbs.
3. This is the one area where I do strongly recommend longer needles as my clinical experience suggests you achieve quicker results.
4. 0.5mm rollers can still achieve results in these cases but work more slowly in this area.
5. Avoiding the sun is usually easier on the thighs than the face and hands and direct sunlight should still be avoided for at least 24 hours and ideally several days.

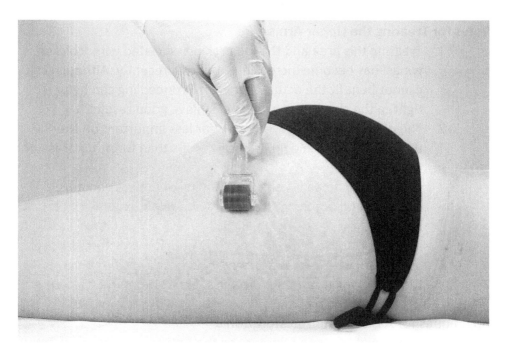
Image 8 – Treating the Thigh Area

Techniques for Treating the Upper Arms

1. Cleanse the area thoroughly using a natural or organic cleanser.
2. Apply the Anti Aging tincture using a cotton pad or simply cleanse with a swab.
3. Select a 0.5mm microneedle roller
4. Apply a vigorous massage to the arm area working upwards towards the chest.
5. Start on the front of the right arm and roll upwards towards the chest across the area being treated. Move gradually across to the back of the arm continuing to roll upwards.
6. Roll perpendicular across the area just treated either from front to back or back to front.
7. Repeat on the left arm.
8. Roll across each area 10-15 times before moving on.
9. Apply the Anti Aging aftercare serum liberally to the area.
10. Follow the aftercare advice and avoid bright sunlight wherever possible for several days. If bright sunlight is unavoidable then high quality SPF 30+ sunscreen should be applied.
11. Continue to apply the Anti Aging aftercare serum twice a day for 2 weeks after treatment.

Notes for Treating the Upper Arms

1. Treating this area and the loose skin associated with 'chicken wings' has become increasingly popular recently. Although it cannot benefit the actual sagging microneedling can help tighten the skin in this area and achieve good results.
2. The direction in which you roll is far less important on the upper arms for achieving clinical results than for other areas of the body.
3. In this case I actually roll against many of the acupuncture channels and opt instead to follow the direction of venous blood return.
4. It is important to only massage upwards towards the trunk so as to work with venous drainage and not damage the valves in the veins which cause blood to pool in the limbs.

Techniques for Assisting Hair Restoration

1. Apply a straight Ginseng tincture or the Anti aging tincture directly to the scalp. Massage this tincture gently into the scalp to ensure full coverage. Home users can skip this step and simply apply the Hair Restoration Spray.
2. Using a dermastamp or microneedle roller start at the front of the hair line in the centre of the head. Work your way backward all the way down to the back of the head.
3. Still working from the front to the back gradually work your way across to the right covering the entire right hand side of the head.
4. Repeat on the left hand side.
5. Only work from front to back as this follows the flow of the acupuncture channels on the head.
6. Next work from the right hand side of the head to the left starting at the front and working your way backwards.
7. Roll or stamp each area 10-15 times.
8. Apply the Hair restoration Spray to the area following treatment. It will take 6-10 pumps of the spray to cover the head. Massage this gently into the scalp.

Notes for Assisting Hair Restoration

1. When treating the scalp the amount of hair remaining on the head influences which needle size you choose. As increasing circulation and transdermal absorption is your main focus here you can use shorter needles than when you are inducing collagen.

2. When a patient has very little hair such as men who have lost the majority of their hair or who are shaving their head then the 0.5mm roller is usually the best length to use. When treating women who having thinning hair but who still have quite long hair in places it is better not to use the roller at all and instead use a dermastamp. This is because longer hair often gets caught in the axel of the roller and is then pulled out. If you do have to use a roller it can help to first wet their hair as it is more likely to sit flat. Only roll in one direction as the change of direction will again ruffle the hair making it more likely to get caught.

3. Keep in mind when using the stamp that it takes more time than the roller. It is also much easier to miss a section so you need to be careful to ensure even coverage.

4. When needling the scalp I first apply an extract of ginseng. This is an herb that was traditionally used topically for hair loss and modern research has shown that it has an inhibitory effect on the testosterone 5α Reductase which is strongly linked to hair loss[13].

5. Clients or home users losing hair will need to understand that 'Hair Restoration' is an on-going issue and generally male clients need to use the products at home on an on-going basis to avoid future hair loss. Female clients suffering temporary post-partum hair loss will not need to use the products on an on-going basis.

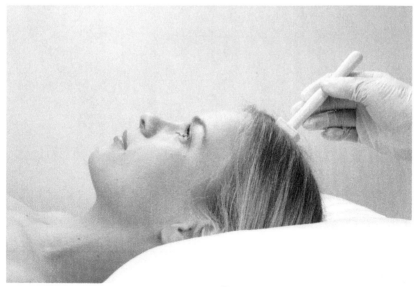

Image 9 – Dermastamp for Hair Restoration

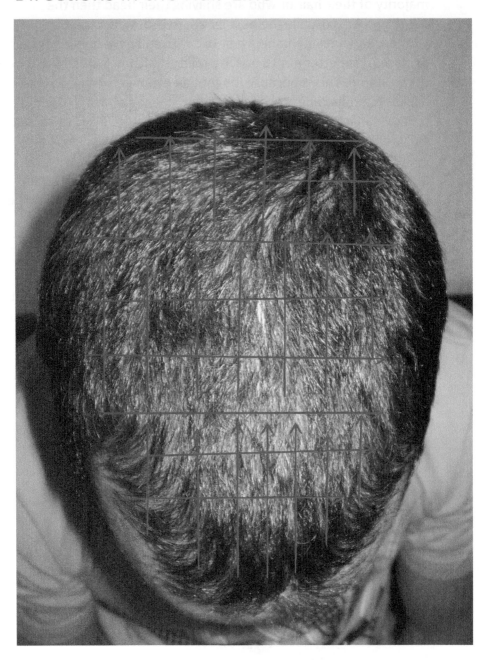

Quick Reference Table

Remember the key ingredients of the tinctures and serums were listed earlier

Condition Being Treated	Microneedle Length	Alcoholic Tincture	Green Tea Oil Aftercare Serum	Direction to Roll In
Anti Aging Facial - includes Collagen Induction, Wrinkles, Thin Skin, Enlarged Pores, Skin Laxity	0.5mm	Anti Aging Tincture	Anti Aging Serum	Upwards and Outwards
UV Damage	0.5mm	Anti Aging Tincture	Anti Aging Serum	Upwards and Outwards
Hands – Anti Aging	0.5mm	Anti Aging Tincture	Anti Aging Serum	Towards the Body and then Across
Hair Loss	1.0mm Or 0.75mm	Anti Aging Tincture	Hair Restoration Spray	Front to Back and then Right to Left
Sagging Upper Arms	0.5mm	Anti Aging Tincture	Anti Aging Serum	Towards the Body and then Across
Age Spots	0.5mm	Anti Aging Tincture	Anti Aging Serum	Dependent on the Location
Redness or Inactive Acne	0.5mm	Clear Skin Tincture	Scar Serum	Upwards and Outwards on the Face.

Non Pustular Rosacea	0.5mm	Clear Skin Tincture	Scar Serum	Upwards and Outwards on the Face.
Hyperpigmentation	0.5mm	Clear Skin Tincture	Scar Serum	Upwards and Outwards on the Face.
Shallow Facial Scars	0.75mm	Scar Tincture	Scar Serum	Upwards and Outwards
Severe Scarring	1.5mm	Scar Tincture	Scar Serum	Dependent on the Location
Stretch Marks	1.5mm	Stretch Mark Tincture	Stretch Mark & Cellulite Serum	Abdomen – Upwards and Outwards Thighs – Upwards and Across
Cellulite	1.5mm	Cellulite Tincture	Stretch Mark & Cellulite Serum	Thighs – Upwards and Across

Chapter 14 - Aftercare

What to Expect?

1. There will normally be redness in the area. This is normal and is a result of the inflammation that causes collagen induction. With a 0.5mm roller this will usually clear within a few hours but can persist for up to 2 days in some cases.
2. You may experience some itchiness in the area due to the release of histamines. This is often worse for those with a history of asthma or sinusitis. In rare cases this can lead to urticarial and you should consult a physician in these cases.
3. Some dry skin may be experienced and the green tea oil is useful to assist this. This dry skin is caused because the moisture barrier of the skin has been breached by the microneedles and is a normal reaction.
4. The skin may feel tender to touch.
5. You may experience an immediate feeling of tightening in the skin. This is because microneedling immediately shortens the elastin fibres so tightening the skin
6. You may also be more sensitive to sunlight straight after treatment. This affect can last for several days. Avoidance of direct sunlight is preferable and if this is not possible SPF 15 or above sunscreen should be applied.
7. In rare cases there may be some bruising or swelling.
8. In rare cases small pustules may form on the skin these should be brought to a clinician or a physician's attention if they persist. They may need to be drained to avoid the formation of scabs that can prevent the absorption of the serum. This is more likely to occur in those suffering from acne scarring.
9. Individuals with darker skin pigmentation may not show the same level of redness and inflammation as lighter skinned individuals however they should follow the same aftercare instructions.

What to Do Following a Treatment?

1. As soon as possible have a shower. Make sure it is not too warm as the skin may be sensitive. Massage the skin gently to remove and residual serum or fluids that may have dried on the skin.
2. Do not have a bath as there is increased risk of contamination from blocked drains.

3. Do not use any skin products on the skin other than those designed to be used with microneedling for 8 hours after treatment. This usually means avoiding moisturisers, make up and shampoo until the next day. Microneedling increases absorption of most products placed on the skin for several hours afterwards and it is important not to use any products that contain potentially toxic ingredients on the skin during this period. As there is no definitive list of ingredients which may be harmful following microneedling it is best to use as few products as possible for the next 24 hours.
4. Direct sunlight should be avoided for around 48 hours following a 0.5mm roller treatment. The period to avoid direct sunlight can be longer with longer microneedles and 14 days if often recommended is using a 1.5mm roller or longer.
5. Where possible avoiding direct sunlight is preferable to sunscreens for the first 24 hours as they can cause adverse skin reactions.
6. Where possible avoid alcohol based products on the skin for 14 days after treatment as they can make the skin feel very dry.
7. If you experience any unexpected adverse reactions please contact your practitioner or seek medical attention.

Anticipated Results Following a Treatment
1. After the first treatment skin will often feel tighter and look fresher.
2. The increase in collagen induction begins within 48 hours of treatment. However it usually takes at least 4 weeks for superior results to be seen.
3. The results will continue to improve for 3-12 months after the treatments as a whole new collagen matrix is formed within the skin.
4. New collagen laid down should last for a period of 5-7 years making microneedling a very long lasting treatment.
5. The collagen induction will usually result in a decreased appearance of lines and wrinkles and an increase in the firmness of the skin.
6. Depending on what is being treated there should also be a reduction in visible scar tissue, reduced signs of UV damage, tightening of the skin, reduced hyperpigmentation, less rosacea, thickening of the skin, reduced skin laxity, increase in scalp hair

growth, a reduction in the signs of stretch marks and an improvement in cellulite.

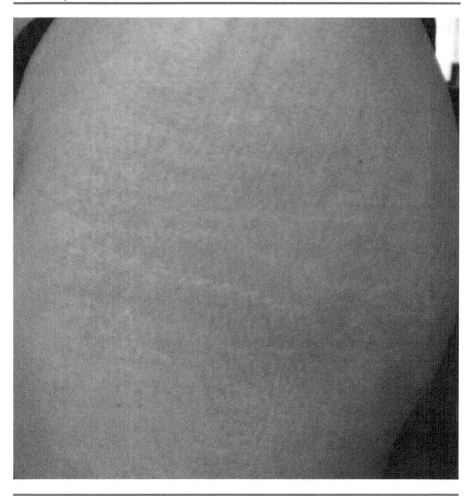

Image 10: The appearance of the skin 10 minutes after treatment. This individual is of Northern Indian origin and how flushed the skin appears varies with different skin types.

Chapter 15 – Comparing Holistic Microneedling to 'Medical Skin Needling'

What is 'Medical Skin Needling'?
It is worth examining in more detail what has become known as 'Medical Skin Needling'. The term medical skin needling has come to be associated with certain practices which are applied to a cosmetic microneedling treatment. These practices are;

1. The use of 1.5mm needles or longer on the face for all purposes.
2. The use of topical vitamin A during the procedure.
3. Excessive bleeding of the skin.
4. The use of topical anaesthetic and in some cases local anaesthetic due to the painful nature of the needling
5. Extensive trauma and long recovery times.

The Benefits of Holistic Microneedling over 'Medical Skin Needling'
1. It has been shown that 0.5mm needles are the smallest that will effectively produce collagen induction. Why use longer needles that cause more structural damage if you are not achieving better results.
2. The use of vitamin A is unnecessary to achieve the results from microneedling which are principally from the induction of collagen. Given that vitamin A has a degree of known toxicity even used topically and dramatically worsens the dryness caused by microneedling there does not seem to be good enough reason to use these products.
3. If using a 0.5mm roller and using the correct technique shown above then most practitioners find it unnecessary to use anaesthetic. Anaesthetic is very useful for some procedures but if it is not needed why expose the skin to it unnecessarily.
4. There is no evidence that bleeding the skin excessively leads to better results and in fact it simply leads to longer recovery times, higher risks of infections and much higher patient dissatisfaction. Many clinicians and all home users are also not set up to deal with large amounts of blood. Even when using the 0.5mm roller you will see the occasional drop of blood but excessive bleeding should be avoided.

5. Long recovery times are never desirable and are simply not necessary if performing microneedling in the ways described in this book.

Does Microneedling Have to be Painful?
The simple answer to this is no, it does not have to be. Due to the use of too longer needles and poor techniques microneedling or skin needling has come to be considered by many as a painful experience. The pain caused by poor practices has been exasperated by a wider community fear of needles and some videos on such sites as You tube showing very bloody and unpleasant treatments.

In clinic I have been practiced consistently for many years using a 0.5mm microneedle roller without ever using topical anaesthetic. Nor has the need for it ever come up. Patients often report the treatments as 'prickly' but rarely report the sensation as painful.

In recent years I have taught hundreds of clinicians our techniques for using the microneedle rollers. In these seminars I teach the use of a 0.5mm and sometimes the 0.75mm roller with no anaesthetic. Clinicians have to practice on each other so they can experience how the treatment feels. The constant feedback has been one of surprise. Most had either heard or been taught elsewhere how painful it would be (often taught the hard way).

More recently I added a question on pain perception to the student feedback form submitted following the seminars. 100% of students have so far submitted the form and so far 91% of 70 students have agreed that the treatment is not painful. Bearing in mind that these treatments are being performed by clinicians using the rollers for the first time these figures are fairly convincing.

The research on this subject is limited but seems to support my findings. In the first item of research microneedle arrays of 0.15mm length were inserted into the skin of 12 subjects and compared to pressing a flat surface against the skin (negative control) and inserting a 26-gauge hypodermic needle into the skin surface (positive control)[72]. Subjects were unable to distinguish between the painless sensation of the flat surface and that caused by microneedles. These needles are shorter than those I recommend so we also need to look at other research.

An article discussing pain perception and the 0.5mm needle length was published in 2007. It showed that microneedles ranging in length between 0.5mm and 0.75mm were perceived as between 10-20 times less painful than a 26 gauge hypodermic needle[73]. A later article was published in 2008 using microneedle lengths from 0.48mm to 1.45mm. These needle lengths were again compared to a 26 gauge hypodermic syringe. The results showed the pain scores varied at between 5-40% of those of the hypodermic syringe with the shorter needles producing the lower scores[74].

This suggests that the 0.48mm (very similar to the 0.5mm needles) produced closer to 5% of the pain of the hypodermic syringe and supports the findings of the previous study. This study also showed statistically that longer microneedles rapidly increase the perception of pain and therefore supports the idea of applying the shortest microneedle that will achieve the results.

This study also produced an interesting result that surprised the researchers. Neither increasing microneedle width nor thickness by 3 fold increased the perception of pain. I have been arguing this for some time that thicker needles are in fact more effective as they do not affect pain levels but are less likely to become blunt or damaged. Blunt and damaged needles definitely do affect the perception of pain as well as causing damage to the skin.

These studies show that very little pain is produced by the shorter microneedles even when using random insertion methods such as those used during this study. By using the correct technique I would suggest you can eliminate even this amount of pain for most people and create a painless microneedling treatment. These studies certainly do not support the idea that anaesthetic is a necessary part of a microneedling treatment.

Chapter 16 - Reusing the Microneedle Roller?

Reusing the microneedle roller refers to reusing the rollers on the same individual repeatedly over a period of time. Microneedle rollers can and should never be reused on different individuals as they cannot be effectively sterilised once used. Any company claiming this does not understand the terminology. We can clean or disinfect a microneedle roller but not sterilise once it has been used.

The 3 Main Issues with Reusing the Roller

1. The first issue is the risk of bacterial infection with reuse. As the roller has previously been in contact with blood it has a higher risk of causing a bacterial infection than a brand new roller. Actually the risk is very low. Despite the huge home use market skin infections are rarely seen. Provided effective cleaning of the roller takes place before and after treatments this is a relatively low risk.

2. The second major issue principally affects clinicians. In many countries it accepted practice to write the clients name in a book and put a number next to it. The number is then written on the used microneedle roller and the roller stored until the clients next visit. To me this is a much larger issue as there is the potential for confusion with another used microneedle roller. Although the risk is small the consequences could be so severe that I do not think this is a risk worth taking. It is not a risk taken with any other needle device used in either cosmetic or medical clinics in most of the Western world.

   This puts clinicians in a difficult position as they must purchase a new roller for every treatment adding to their costs while less conscientious clinicians can achieve higher profit margins by reusing the rollers. This can however be a reputational asset. There are many clients in the market who would not be interested in using any form of needle at home and would expect their clinician to remove any device containing needles from tamper evident packaging in front of them. This is why cosmetic clinics carrying higher quality brands of microneedle rollers and other products can always command a premium for their services.

3. If a clinic is located in a country where it is legal and your insurance will cover the practice of reusing microneedle rollers or you are an individual using a home use roller then there is a third issue to be dealt with. Over time the needles can become blunt or bent. It is often hard to see a blunt or bent needle on visual inspection. The first signs of blunt of damaged needles are they feel like they are dragging or catching on the skin. This is a sure sign that the roller needs replacing.

Some roller designs are better for reusing than others. Generally the rollers with the flat handles that sit horizontally in cases are less easy to damage as you can get the rollers in and out of the case easily without bumping them and the case protects the needles between treatments. Cylindrical handle rollers that arrive in tube packaging are harder to reuse as every time you put them in or out you have to be very careful not to let the roller touch the side of the tube as this damages all the needles along the edge of the roller.

Ultimately if you are reusing the microneedle roller all rollers will need replacing after a period of time. You can lessen how often a roller is replaced by buying higher quality microneedle rollers from a reputable supplier. When it comes to microneedle rollers there is some truth in the saying 'you get what you pay for'.

Cleaning the Rollers
If you are reusing the microneedle rollers then it is important to have an effective cleaning process. There are a wide variety of methods advertised for cleaning the roller. Despite this the recorded infection rate with use of microneedling rollers in extremely low indicating that the rollers are fairly safe under a variety of conditions.

Below is a simple process that can be followed to clean the roller directly after use.

1. Rinse the roller under warm running water. This step becomes more important if using longer needles and more invasive techniques as more blood is produced and attaches to the drum of the roller.
2. Apply isopropyl alcohol of at least 70% to disinfect the roller. Notice the word is disinfect not sterilise as this is not possible with

any microneedle roller. This can be done in 2 ways. It can be sprayed repeatedly with an isopropyl alcohol spray for several minutes making sure the roller is thoroughly soaked. Alternatively it can be soaked in alcohol for 30 minutes in a plastic cup on a cotton wool ball. Theoretically this is more effective but has a higher chance of damaging the needles and ruining the roller.

3. Prior to the next treatment again spray the roller with the isopropyl alcohol spray thoroughly. The alcohol evaporates rapidly, however you still need to allow several minutes from when the roller is sprayed before using the roller.

4. This is the simplest technique available and as stated above cleans but does not sterilise the roller meaning it cannot be used on other people only the one individual.

Another popular technique is to soak the roller in water containing a denture tablet. Denture tablets usually contain persulfates which can cause a variety of allergic reactions[75]. This should not be a large risk with the rollers as they should be rinsed thoroughly afterwards but I would still avoid any unnecessary chemicals as part of a holistic approach to microneedling.

The final technique which can be practiced is the use of colloidal silver which is very effective for disinfecting metal and is very affordable for home users. It can be substituted for the use of alcohol in the above process.

Chapter 17 - Complimentary Treatments

As part of my approach to holistic microneedling I incorporate cosmetic techniques from my training in Traditional Chinese Medicine. The use of the Jade roller is one of the simplest techniques that can be combined with the microneedle roller to create a truly holistic treatment. It is quick to learn, effective and feels wonderful on the skin.

What are Jade Rollers?

As the name suggests jade rollers are small rollers made of solid jade crystal. Jade is traditionally the stone of wealth and beauty in China. Jade rollers were an essential part of the cosmetic regime of every wealthy woman in ancient China and have been found in tombs dating back around 2,000 years ago indicating the longevity of their use. They were traditionally kept wrapped in silk providing another indicator of how highly they were valued.

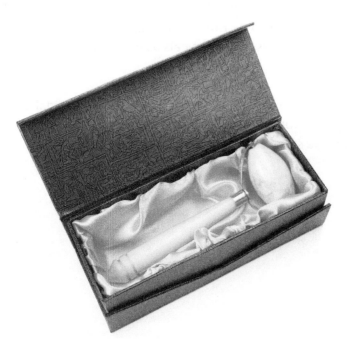

Image 11: A Jade Roller in its Traditional Silk Lined Box

What are Jade Rollers Used For?

Traditionally they were used to flatten wrinkles on the face and clear fluid congestion. Jade is an unusual semiprecious stone in that it remains cold while in contact with the skin and this allows it to help close the pores and tighten the skin. In modern scientific understanding their most useful function is that they increase lymphatic drainage.

Increasing Lymphatic Drainage
Here we are referring to the interstitial fluid or the fluid that resides within the tissues. This fluid is responsible for providing cell nutrition and removing waste products and toxins. The lymphatic system has no pump to keep the lymph circulating and instead relies on muscle contraction. When this system does not function correctly there is a build-up of fluid in the tissues which can manifest as swelling and fluid retention in an area.

The lymphatic system responds very well to manual therapy. This can be done in a variety of ways, one of the easiest and cheapest being with a jade roller massage.

By improving lymphatic circulation you can provide improved nutrition to the cells in the epidermis and dermis. You can also increase the removal of waste products.

This is very useful in combination with microneedling as the micro trauma caused by the needles requires good nutrition to heal and the healing process creates a variety of waste products that need to be removed from the area.

How to Use the Jade Roller
Jade rollers are quick and easy to use. They are also excellent to use on sensitive areas such as the eyes and neck.

The jade rollers are rolled across the face in an upward and outward direction. They can be applied immediately using the following steps.

1. Start all techniques on the right side of the face and repeat on the left hand side afterwards.
2. Unlike the microneedle roller you can use long smooth strokes.
3. Roll gently up the throat on both sides and the middle.
4. From the chin roll out along the jaw line.
5. Gradually move upwards rolling the entire cheek area in an outwards direction.
6. From the edge of the nose roll laterally under the eyes.
7. Next roll upwards across the entire cheek

8. From the lateral corner of the eyes roll outwards across the crow's feet.
9. From the centre of the forehead roll outwards laterally.
10. From the tip of the nose roll upwards to the hair line.
11. Continue to roll upwards across the entire forehead.
12. You can use the diagram of the microneedle roller use on the face to ensure you are rolling in the right direction.
13. You can also watch videos about the jade rollers on our You Tube Channel at http://www.youtube.com/user/whitelotusantiaging

Home users can use the roller after a microneedle treatment. They are fantastic at this point at cooling the skin that can feel a little inflamed and hot after microneedling.

Clinicians are better advised to use the jade rollers before the microneedling if they plan to reuse the jade roller. If used before the microneedling process they can be cleaned and reused. As they are not porous some clinicians have argued that they can be used after the microneedling and that they can be sterilised by the use of isopropyl alcohol and a UV sanitizer. This still presents a small risk that I believe is best avoided.

Clinicians can also experiment with using 2 jade rollers simultaneously. This is extremely luxurious and relaxing for the client which is great if the client is at all nervous about the microneedle treatment.

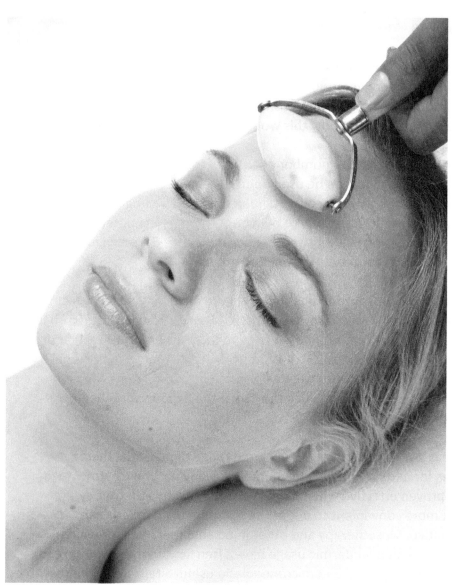

Image 12: The Jade Roller in Use

Chapter 18 - The Future of Microneedling

Currently the use of microneedling is focused on two specific areas, cosmetic use and increasing the absorption of pharmaceutical drugs. This dual focus is creating an impetus for research which is allowing us to learn more and more about how this wonderful therapy works.

There are an increasing number of areas of the body that the microneedling roller can be used upon to achieve cosmetic results. The use of microneedling for collagen induction is also being embraced by many clinicians to assist severe post burn trauma. The potential of microneedling for a variety of other cosmetic uses based on inducting collagen will undoubtedly continue to grow.

The increased absorption possible with microneedling has only just begun to be explored. A recent review of the evidence strongly suggests that microneedle vaccines are more effective than either intramuscular or subcutaneous injections[23]. It is now believed by many in the industry that most future vaccines will be delivered by microneedles and a range of other possibilities to reduce the use of the hypodermic needle are being researched.

There is also a huge largely unexplored range of potential therapeutic usages for natural and holistic therapies. Many natural treatments that have proven effective when delivered through a hypodermic syringe may find it more convenient to adopt the microneedling roller as an alternative. Mesotherapy and other injectable therapies for which regulations on hypodermic usage have often limited their widespread distribution may also find microneedles a useful alternative. The research on vaccines above should be of great interest to the practitioners of mesotherapy who often use homeopathic preparations for similar purposes.

In a variety of fields the potential increase in transdermal absorption available with microneedling may open up whole new ideas about product administration.

Hopefully we can approach this with more imagination to engage new ideas and then provide the research and practice to ensure their safety and effectiveness.

Before and After Photos

Some of these were taken in our clinic and others have been provided by our students or patients.

Before

After

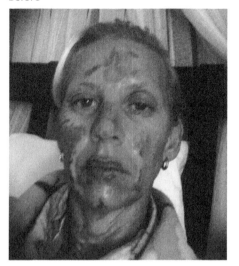 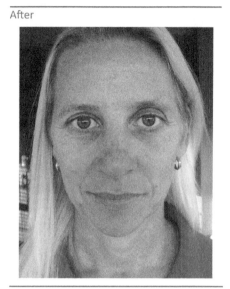

A client who suffered severe burn scars from a grass fire. The early photos show her still in the healing stage. She was concerned about the scarring that was developing. She began treatment very soon afterwards. It can be seen in the after photo taken by her 3 months later that her very fair skin shows virtually no scarring. She used the 0.5mm roller with a green tea oil scar serum once a week for the entire period.

Before

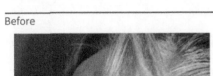

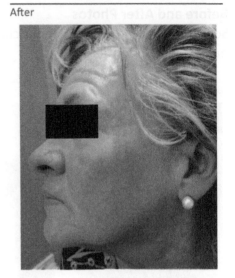

This Patient received a series of anti aging microneedle treatments over several months. Photo donated by Helen Kirby

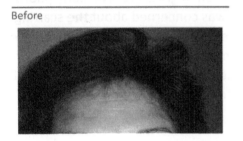

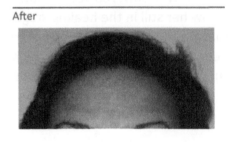

This 55 year old patient received 6 microneedle treatments using a 0.5mm roller over a 15 week period.

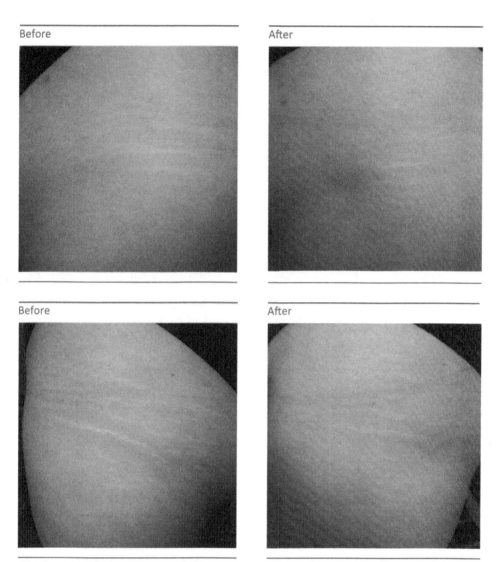

Before

After

Before

After

Both sets of photos are of the same patient who received 3 treatments using a 1.5mm roller, and the Stretch mark tincture. She used the Aftercare serum at home during the period.

Before After

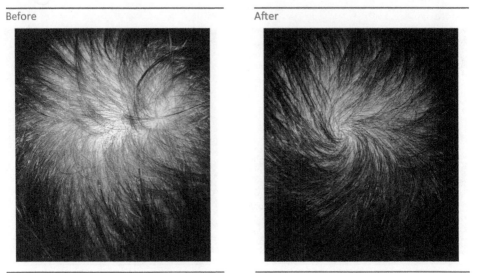

A 35 year old man after using a 1.0mm dermastamp and the Hair Restoration spray over a period of 6 weeks

Before After

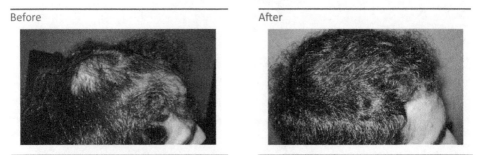

Client in his mid 30's before and after 3 months of using the 1.0mm microneedling roller with the restoration spray.

References

1. Disegi, J.A. & Eschbach, L. (2000). Stainless steel in bone surgery. *Injury,* 31, Supp 4:2-6.

2. Gill, H. S., Denson, D. D., Burris, B. A. & Prausnitz, M. R. (2008). Effect of microneedle design on pain in human subjects. *Clin J Pain.* 24(7), 585–594.

3. Zhang, Q. & and Zhu, L. (1996). Meridional Cosmetology: Report of 300 Cases with Discussion of Underlying Mechanism. *The International Journal of Clinical Acupuncture.* 7(4), 401-405.

4. Henry, S. McAllister, D.V. Allen, M.G. Prausnitz, M.R. (1998). Microfabricated microneedles: a novel approach to transdermal drug delivery. *J Pharm Sci.* Aug87(8), 922-925.

5. Orentreich, D.S. Orentreich, N. (1995). Subcutaneous incisionless (subcision) surgery for the correction of depressed scars and wrinkles. *Dermatol Surg.* Jun21(6). 543-549.

6. Fernandes, D. (1996). Upper lip line treatment. *Paper presented at the ISAPS Conference.* Taipei, Taiwan.

7. Badram, M. M., Kuntsche, J. & Fahr, A. (2009). Skin penetration enhancement by a microneedle device (Dermaroller®) in vitro: Dependency on needle size and applied formulation. *European journal of pharmaceutical sciences.* 3 6, 511–523.

8. Midwood, K.S., Williams, L.V., Schwarzbauer, J.E. (2004). Tissue repair and the dynamics of the extracellular matrix. *The International Journal of Biochemistry & Cell Biology* 36 (6), 1031–1037.

9. Anastassakis, K. (2005). The Dermaroller™ Series. Retrieved July, 30, 2011 from http://www.oniskai.com/pdf/Anastassakis_Article.pdf

10. Setterfield, L. (2010). The concise guide to Dermal Needling (Medical Edition). Whangaparaoa: Virtual Beauty Corporation Ltd.

11. Yano, K., Brown, L. F. & Detmar, M. (2001). Control of Hair Growth and Follicle Size by VEGF-Mediated Angiogenesis JCl. *Journal of Clinical Investigations.* 107(4), 409-417.

12. Takakura, N., Yoshida, H., Kunisada, T., Nishikawa, S. & Nishikawa1, S. (1996). Involvement of Platelet-Derived Growth Factor Receptor-alpha in Hair Canal Formation. *Journal of Investigative Dermatology.* 107, 770–777.

13. Murata, K., Takeshita, F., Samukawa, K., Tani, T. & Matsuda, H. (2011). Effects of Ginseng Rhizome and Ginsenoside Ro on Testosterone 5a-Reductase and Hair Re-growth in Testosterone-treated Mice. *Phytother Res.* Jan 26(1), 48-53.

14. Alberti, I., Kalia, Y.N., Naik, A., Bonny, J.D. & Guy, R.H., (2001). Effect of ethanol and isopropyl myristate on the availability of topical terbinafine in human stratum corneum, in vivo. *Int. J. Pharm.* 219, 11–19.

15. Barry, B.W. (1987). Mode of action of penetration enhancers in human skin. *J. Control. Rel.* 6, 85–97.

16. Williams, A.C. & Barry, B.W. (2004). Penetration enhancers. *Adv.Drug Deliv. Rev.* 56, 603–618.

17. Kalia, Y.N., Naik, A., Garrison, J. & Guy, R.H. (2004). Iontophoretic drug delivery. *Adv. Drug Deliv. Rev.* 56, 619–658.

18. Merino, G., Kalia, Y.N. & Guy, R.H. (2003). Ultrasound-enhanced transdermal transport. *J. Pharm. Sci.* 92, 1125–1137.

19. Mitragotri, S. & Kost, J. (2004). Low-frequency sonophoresis. A review. *Adv. Drug Deliv. Rev.* 56, 589–601.

20. Sen, A., Daly, M.E. & Hui, S.W. (2002). Transdermal insulin delivery using lipid enhanced electroporation. *BBA,* 1564, 5–8.

21. Denet, A.R., Vanbever, R. & Preat, V. (2004). Skin electroporation for transdermal and topical delivery. *Adv. Drug Deliv. Rev.* 56, 659–674.

22. Matriano, J.A., Cormier, M., Johnson, J., Young, W. A., Buttery, M., Nyam, K., Daddona, P., (2002). Macroflux® Microprojection Array Patch Technology: A New and Efficient Approach for Intracutaneous Immunization. *Pharmaceutical research.* 19(1), 63-70.

23. Prausnitz, M. R., Mikszta, J. A., Cormier, M. & Andrianov, A. K. (2009). Microneedle-based vaccines. *Curr Top Microbiol Immunol,* 333, 369-393.

24. Ellner, P. D. (1998). Smallpox: Gone but not forgotten. *Infection.* Sep-Oct, 26(5), 263-269.

25. Cormier, M., Johnson, B., Ameri, M., Nyam, K., Libiran, L., Zhang, D.D., Daddona, P. (2004). Transdermal delivery of desmopressin using a coated microneedle array patch system. *J. Control. Rel.* 97, 503–511.

26. McAllister, D.V., Wang, P.M., Davis, S.P., Park, J.H., Canatella, P.J., Allen, M.G., Prausnitz, M.R. (2003). Microfabricated needles fortransdermal delivery of macromolecules and nanoparticles: fabrication methods and transport studies. *PNAS* 100, 13755–13760.

27. Cristina, C., Abad Casintahan, F. (2011)Transepidermal Delivery of Tranexamic Acid vs. Placebo using the Dermaroller in the Treatment of Melasma. *Presentation at the Phillipine Dermatological Society for the Jose R. Reyes Memorial Medical Center.*

28. Yoon, J., Son, T., Choi, E., Choi, B., Nelson, J. S. & Jung, B. (2008). Enhancement of optical skin clearing efficacy using a microneedle roller. Journal of Biomedical Optics 13(2), 021103.

29. 4-Schwartz et al, 2006, internet paper. Abstract reflections about COLLAGEN-INDUCTION-THERAPY (CIT) A Hypothesis for the Mechanism of Action of Collagen Induction Therapy (CIT) using Micro-Needles; 1st edition February 2006. 2nd revision January 2007 Horst Liebl

30. Aust, M. C., Fernandes, D., Kolokythas, P., Kaplan, H. M, & Vogt, P. M. (2008). Percutaneous Collagen induction therapy an alternative treatment for scars, wrinkles and skin laxity. *Plast Reconstr Surg.* 121, 1421-1429.

31. Aust, M. C., Reimers, K., Kaplan, H. M., Stahl, F,. Repenning, C., Scheper, T., Jahn, S., Schwaiger, N., Ipaktchi, R., Redeker, J., Altintas, M. A. & Vogt, P. M. (2011). Percutaneous collagen inductioneregeneration in place of cicatrisation? *Journal of Plastic, Reconstructive & Aesthetic Surgery.* 64, 97-107

32. Aust, M.C., Reimers, K., Repenning, C., Stahl, F., Jahn, S., Guggenheim, M., Schwaiger, N., Gohritz, A. & Vogt, P. M. (2008). Percutaneous collagen induction: minimally invasive skin rejuvenation without risk of hyperpigmentation-fact or fiction? *Plast Reconstr Surg.* 122(5), 1553-63.

33. Majid, I.(2009). Micro needling Therapy in Atrophic Facial Scars: An Objective Assessment. *J Cutan Aesthet Surg.* Jan–Jun 2(1), 26–30.

34. Aust, M. C., Knobloch, K., Reimers, K., Redeker, J., Ipaktchi, R., Altintas, M.A., Gohritz, A., Schwaiger, N. & Vogt, P. M. (2010). Percutaneous collagen induction therapy: an alternative treatment for burn scars. *Burns.* Sep 36(6), 836-43. Epub 2010 Jan 13.

35. Aust, M.C., Vogt, P. M. & Knobloch, K. (2010). Percutaneous collagen induction therapy as a therapeutic option for striae distensae. *Plast Reconstr Surg.* Oct 126(4), 219e-220e.

36. Aust, M., Knobloch, K., Gohritz, A., Vogt, P. M. & Fernandes, D.(2010). Percutaneous Collagen Induction Therapy for Hand Rejuvenation. *Plast Reconstr Surg*. Oct 126(4), 203e-204e.

37. Kim, S. E., Lee, J. H., Kwon, H. B., Ahn, B. J. & Lee, A. Y. (2011). Greater collagen deposition with the micro needle therapy system than with intense pulsed light. *Dermatol Surg*. Mar 37(3), 336-341

38. You, S. K., Noh, Y. W., Park, H. H., Han, M., Lee, S.S., Shin, S.C. & Cho, C.W. (2010). Effect of applying modes of the polymer microneedle-roller on the permeation of L-ascorbic acid in rats. *J Drug Target*. Jan 18(1), 15-20.

39. FDA (2008). Early Communication about an Ongoing Safety Review of Botox and Botox Cosmetic (Botulinum toxin Type A) and Myobloc (Botulinum toxin Type B). Retrieved January, 10, 2012. From http://www.fda.gov/Drugs/DrugSafety/PostmarketDrugSafetyInformationforPatientsand Providers/DrugSafetyInformationforHeathcareProfessionals/ucm070366.htm

40. Lyer, S., Carranza, D., Kolodney, M., MacGregor, D., Chipps, L. &Soriano, T., (2007). Evaluation of procollagen I deposition after intense pulsed light treatments at varying parameters in a porcine model. *J Cosmet Laser Ther* 9, 75–78.

41. Luo, D., Cao, Y., Wu, D., Xu, Y., Chen, B. & Xue, Z. (2009). Impact of intense pulse light irradiation on BALB/c mouse skin-in vivo study on collagens, matrix metalloproteinases and vascular endothelial growth factor. *Lasers Med Sci*, 24, 101–108.

42. Wang, P.M., Cornwell, M., Hill, J.& Prausnitz, M.R. (2006). Precise microinjection into skin using hollow microneedles. *J. Invest. Dermatol*. 126, 1080–1087.

43. Wermeling, D.P., Banks, S.L., Hudson, D.A., Gill, H.S., Gupta, J.,Prausnitz, M.R. & Stinchcomb, A.L. (2008). Microneedles permit transdermal delivery of a skin-impermeant medication to humans. *PNAS*, 2058–2063.

44. Silverman, A.K., Ellis, C. N. & Voorhees, J. J. (1987). Hypervitaminosis A Syndrome: A Paradigm of Retinoid Side Effects. *The Journal of the American Academy of Dermatology*. 16(5), 1027-1039.

45. Lips, P. (2003). Hypervitaminosis A and fractures. *N Engl J Med*. 348(4),1927–1928.

46. Schwarz, K. W., Mary, M. D., Murray, T., Sylora, R., Sohn, R. L. & Dulchavsky, S. A. (2002). Augmentation of Wound Healing with Translation Initiation Factor eIF4E mRNA. *Journal of Surgical Research*. 103(2). 175-182.

47. Packer, L., (1994). Vitamin E is Nature's Master Antioxidant. *Science & Medicine*, 1(1), 54-63.

48. Burton, G. W., Traber, M. G., Acuff, R.V., Walters, D. N., Kayden, H., Hughes, L. & Ingold, K. U. (1998). Human plasma and tissue alpha-tocopherol concentrations in response to supplementation with deuterated natural and synthetic vitamin E. *Am J Clin Nutr*. Apr 67(4), 669-684.

49. Dairy House. (2011). Vitamin A Palmitate. Retrieved December, 12, 2011 from http://www.dairy-house.com/index.php?p=67 vitamin A production

50. Dictionary.com. Natural Definition. Retrieved January,10, 2012 from http://dictionary.reference.com/browse/natural

51. Lee, J., Jung, E., Lee, J., Huh, S., Kim, J., Park, M... & Park, D. J. (2007). Panax ginseng induces human Type I collagen synthesis through activation of Smad signalling. *Ethnopharmacol*. Jan 3, 109(1), 29-34.

52. Cho, S., Won, C. H., Lee, D. H., Lee, M. J., Lee, S., So, S.H... & Chung, J. H. J. (2009). Red ginseng root extract mixed with Torilus fructus and Corni fructus improves facial

wrinkles and increases type I procollagen synthesis in human skin: a randomized, double-blind, placebo-controlled study. *Med Food*. Dec, 12(6), 1252-1259.

53. Kim, D. W., Eum, W. S., Jang, S. H., Yoon, C. S., Choi, H. S., Choi, S.H. & Choi, S. Y. (2010).Ginsenosides enhance the transduction of tat-superoxide dismutase into mammalian cells and skin. *Mol Cells*. Dec 31, 16(3), 402-406.

54. Lee, J. H., Shim, J. S., Chung, M. S., Lim, S. T. & Kim, K. H. (2009). Inhibition of pathogen adhesion to host cells by polysaccharides from Panax ginseng. *Biosci Biotechnol Biochem*. Jan, 73(1), 209-212.

55. Chen, L. (2005). Use of single component Camellia oil for treatment of scald with no scar left. Famiing Zhuanli Shenqing Gongkai Shuomingshu (p.4) Peop. Rep. China.

56. Chen, Y. H. (2007). Physiochemical properties and bioactivities of tea seed (Camellia oleifera) oil, Clemson Univeristy. Retrieved August, 8, 2012 from http://proquest.umi.com/pqdlink?Ver=1&Exp=08-29-2017&FMT=7&DID=1335360001&RQT=309&attempt=1&cfc=1

57. Hou, R. Y., Wan, X. C. & Wu, H. P. (2006). Preliminary Studies on antimicrobial action of tea saponin. *Food Sci*. 27(1), 51-54.

58. Katiyar, S. K. (2003). Skin photoprotection by green tea: antioxidant and immunomodulatory effects. *Curr Drug Targets Immune Endocr Metabol Disord*. Sep. 3(3), 234-42.

59. Thring, T. S., Hili, P. & Naughton, D. P. (2009). Anti-collagenase, anti-elastase and anti-oxidant activities of extracts from 21 plants. *BMC Complement Altern Med*. Aug 4, 9, 27.

60. Yusuf, N., Irby, C., Katiyar, S. K. & Elmets. C. A. (2007). Review article - Photoprotective effects of green tea polyphenols. *Photodermatol Photoimmunol Photomed*. 23, 48–56.

61. Elmets, C. A., Singh, D., Tubesing, K., Matsui, M., Katiyar, S. & Mukhtar, H. (2001). Cutaneous photoprotection from ultraviolet injury by green tea polyphenols. *J Am Acad Dermatol*. Mar, 44(3), 425-432.

62. Pajonk, F., Riedisser, A., Henke, M., McBride, W. H. & Fiebich, B. (2006). The effects of tea extracts on proinflammatory signalling. *BMC Med*. Dec 1,4,28.

63. Mahmood, T. Akhtar, N., Khan, B. A., Khan, H. M. S. & Saeed, T. (2011). Outcomes of 3% Green Tea Emulsion on Skin Sebum Production in Male Volunteers. BJBMS. 10(3), 260-264.

64. Elsaie, M. L., Abdelhamid, M. F., Elsaaiee, L. T. & Emam, H. M. (2009). The efficacy of topical 2% green tea lotion in mild-to-moderate acne vulgaris. *J Drugs Dermatol*. Apr, 8(4), 358-364.

65. Larsson, S. C., Åkesson, A., Bergkvist, L. & Wolk, A. (2010). Multivitamin use and breast cancer incidence in a prospective cohort of Swedish women. *Am J Clin Nutr* May.

66. Klein, E. A., Thompson, I. M., Tangen, C. M., Crowley, J. J., Lucia, M. S., Goodman, P. J., & Baker, L. H. (2011). Vitamin E and the Risk of Prostate Cancer: Results of The Selenium and Vitamin E Cancer Prevention Trial (SELECT). *JAMA*. 306(14), 1549-1556.

67. Pitchford, P. (2002). Healing with Whole Foods: Asian Traditions and Modern Nutrition. North Atlantic Books, California.

68. Tokusoglu, O. & Unal, M.K. (2003). Biomass Nutrient Profiles of Three Microalgae: Spirulina platensis, Chlorella vulgaris, and Isochrisis galbana. *Journal of Food Science*, 68(4).

69. Donnelly, R. F., Singh, T. R. R., Tunney, M. M., Morrow, D. I. J., McCarron, P. A., O'Mahony, C. & Woolfson, A. D. (2009). Microneedle Arrays Allow Lower Microbial

Penetration Than Hypodermic Needles In Vitro. *Pharm Res*. November 26(11), 2513–2522.

70. Reichmanis, M., Marino, A. A. & Becker, R. O. (1977). Laplace Plane Analysis of Transient
Impedance Between Acupuncture Points Li-4 and Li-12. *Biomedical Engineering, IEEE Transactions*. 24 (4), 402-405.

71. Darras, J. C., Vernejoul, P. & Albarede, P. (1992). Nuclear Medicine and Acupuncture: A study on the migration of Radioactive Tracers after Injection at Acupuncture Points. *American Journal of Acupuncture*. 20, (3), 243-256.

72. Kaushik, S., Hord, A. H., Denson, D. D., McAllister, D. V., Smitra, S., Allen, M. G. & Prausnitz, M. R. (2001). Lack of pain associated with microfabricatedmicroneedles. *Anesth Analg*. Feb,92(2), 502-504.

73. Gill, H. S. & Prausnitz, M. R. (2007). Does Needle Size Matter? *Journal of Diabetes Science and Technology*. 1(5).

74. Gill, H. S., Denson, D., Burris, B. A. & Prausnitz, M. R. (2008). Effect of microneedle design on pain in human subjects. *Clin J Pain*. 24(7). 585-594.

75. Burhenne, M., (2010). The Disturbing Ingredient Hidden in Your Denture Cleanser. Retrieved January, 12, 2012 from, http://askthedentist.com/the-disturbing-ingredient-hidden-in-your-denture-cleanser/

Resources

To learn more about the products, upcoming seminars and educational opportunities with Anthony you can visit the following websites. You can also subscribe to his monthly email which provides a range of on-going articles about microneedling and the beauty secrets of the Far East.

www.whitelotusantiaging.com
www.whitelotusantiaging.co.uk
www.whitelotus.com.au

For a range of educational videos please visit the following website.

www.youtube.com/user/whitelotusantiaging

To keep up to date with a range of educational and industry articles on the White Lotus blog and social media pages please visit the following sites.

www.facebook.com/whitelotusantiaging
www.twitter.com/Whitelotusshop
www.whitelotusantiaging.wordpress.com

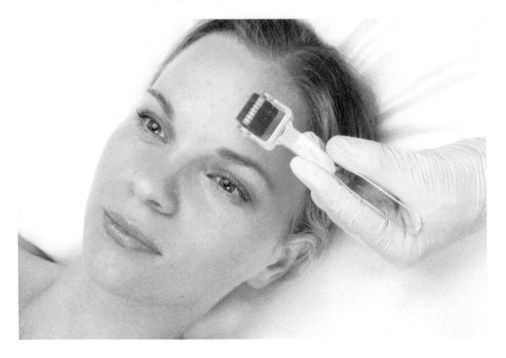

CPSIA information can be obtained at www.ICGtesting.com
Printed in the USA
BVOW10s1054310114

343354BV00002BA/5/P

9 780755 214921